BIOTECHNOLOGY

SCIENCE, ENGINEERING, AND ETHICAL CHALLENGES
FOR THE TWENTY-FIRST CENTURY

Frederick B. Rudolph and Larry V. McIntire, *Editors*

JOSEPH HENRY PRESS
Washington, D.C.   1996

JOSEPH HENRY PRESS • 2101 Constitution Avenue, N.W. • Washington, D.C. 20418

The Joseph Henry Press, an imprint of the National Academy Press, was created with the goal of making books on science, technology, and health more widely available to professionals and the public. Joseph Henry was one of the founders of the National Academy of Sciences and a leader of early American science.

Library of Congress Cataloging-in-Publication Data

Biotechnology : science, engineering, and ethical challenges for the
   21st century / Frederick B. Rudolph and Larry V. McIntire, editors.
      p.   cm.
   Includes bibliographical references and index.
   ISBN 0-309-05282-3
   1. Biotechnology. 2. Biotechnology—Social aspects. I. Rudolph,
Frederick B. II. McIntire, Larry V.
TP248.2.B574   1996
660'.6—dc20   95-44203
                                                  CIP

Dedication

Preface

... [H]umanity is always mistrustful of any radical change, especially so in any field that touches their feelings and instincts. All large biological discoveries are bound to affect human feelings and instincts, and so they will always by a great proportion of mankind be greeted as impious, immoral and indecent.

Julian Huxley, Professor of Biology, Rice University, 1924

[Biotechnology is defined as] techniques that use living organisms to make or modify products, improve plants or animals, and develop micro-organisms for specific purposes.

Definition in use by the National Research Council, 1994

Genetically engineered food, gene therapy, DNA fingerprinting: these are the "sound bite" phrases that define the extent of many people's knowledge of biotechnology as the twenty-first century approaches. Yet biotechnology promises to alter people's lives as radically in the next century as did electricity, telecommunications, and the automobile in the twentieth century.

During the past two decades rapid advances in biotechnology have sparked both great interest and intense debate among scientists and non-scientists alike. This volume is intended to increase awareness and stimulate discussion of both the great opportunities and the difficult challenges that advances in biotechnology present for science and for society.

Biotechnology is first and foremost a set of scientific discoveries and techniques that make it possible to manipulate the basic building blocks of life: DNA molecules and genes. This technology holds the promise of curing disease, repairing environmental damage, and improving the quality and quantity of agricultural production.

Biotechnology is also an industry that had $6 billion in annual sales in 1993 and is growing rapidly, attracting millions of dollars in investment capital and employing thousands of people.

Many people perceive biotechnology as a threat: not only a threat to accepted ways of being, doing, and working, but also an affront to basic moral values. Tinkering with the genetic makeup of living things (especially human beings) is, in the eyes of many, simply wrong. End of discussion.

Except that it isn't the end of the discussion. Biotechnology will not go away if people shut their eyes to it. It is a reality that will significantly affect how individuals live, work, and make decisions about family, health care, and the future.

Nowhere are the opportunities and challenges of biotechnology thrown into sharper relief than in health care. Therapeutic proteins such as insulin, Factor VIII, and human growth hormone are now being manufactured by recombinant DNA technology. Gene therapy experiments have been approved for the treatment of patients with enzyme deficiencies, inherited high blood cholesterol, arthritis, cancer, and other diseases.

Skin, cartilage, blood vessels, and other body tissues are being "grown" in the laboratory. If such tissue engineering can be made to work on a large scale, it may eventually be unnecessary to obtain tissues and organs from human donors for transplantation.

Scientists have succeeded in identifying genes associated with cystic fibrosis, Huntington's disease, breast and colon cancer, and other disorders, making it possible to identify people at high risk for these conditions years before they develop any symptoms. This capability raises enormous questions: Who has access to an individual's genetic information? How might prospective parents react when told that the fetus the woman is carrying has the gene for a devastating illness? Are all the discoveries and techniques of biotechnology necessarily beneficial to society?

Such disturbing questions lead some people to lash out at scientists: "Why can't they leave well enough alone? There are some things we are better off not knowing." Despite the many benefits that science has brought to modern life, and despite (or perhaps because of) the fact that the pace of scientific discovery has never been more rapid, public confidence in science is at a low ebb.

In addition to questions about the societal impact of biotechnology, there are many unresolved issues related to the means by which the products of biotechnology move from the laboratory to the commercial marketplace. Although at first glance these issues appear to be purely pragmatic, a closer look reveals them to be quite complex because they involve questions of values, organizational culture, and public policy.

How much freedom should scientists have to pursue basic, curiosity-driven research? When a private company supports research, how much control should it have over the dissemination of the results of that research? What is the best way to ensure that worthwhile new technologies are developed commercially? Who will make decisions about the safety, efficacy, and cost-effectiveness of new technologies?

Scientists, constrained by funding limitations and pressures to collaborate with industry and to conduct more research that is targeted to specific objectives, worry about maintaining the integrity and vitality of the research enterprise. Biotechnology company executives face a different set of constraints: The commercial development of a biotechnology product involves significant investment risk. Many difficulties are inherent in the manufacture on a large scale of products based on living organisms. Even if these difficulties can be overcome, a stringent, costly regulatory process (intended to safeguard public health) means that many products that undergo testing may ultimately fail to be approved for marketing.

In one way or another, all of these issues touch on what is arguably the central burning issue of U.S. public policy in the 1990s: the proper role and responsibilities of government. Scientists, the biotechnology industry, and the public all have different and often conflicting expectations of government. Can government simultaneously promote scientific research and innovation (as scientists want), encourage the growth of an industry that benefits the economy (as the biotechnology industry wants), and protect public health and individual privacy (as the public wants)?

This thorny set of complex and interrelated concerns formed the backdrop to a conference organized by Rice University's Institute of Biosciences and Bioengineering in the spring of 1994. This book is a product of the discussions that took place at that conference, which brought a distinguished group of scientists, physicians, ethicists, engineers, attorneys, entrepreneurs, and policymakers together to discuss the scientific, engineering, and ethical challenges presented by biotechnology.

The three-day conference was designed to interweave discussions of scientific and ethical issues because the organizers felt that these two sets of issues are too often rigidly separated. The variety of perspectives represented by the conference speakers reflects the convergence of disciplines that is a hallmark of the biotechnological revolution.

This crossdisciplinary bent is also reflected in the book, which includes, for example, a chapter by Daniel E. Koshland, Jr., distinguished former editor-in-chief of *Science* magazine, on the ethical issues raised by biotechnology. A chapter on the investigation of scientific misconduct is contributed by lawyer Barbara Mishkin. Michael Shuler, professor of chemical engineering at Cornell University, provides an engineer's perspective on the development of biopharmaceuticals.

The book is organized into five sections. Part 1 focuses on basic research in biotechnology, including an overview of recombinant DNA technology, which launched the biotechnological revolution in the 1970s. These chapters orient the reader by outlining the history of biotechnology, describing the current state of the art, and hinting at the challenges that these advances present for society.

Part 2 spotlights current and promising future applications of biotechnology in health care and environmental restoration, delineating both the enormous potential of the technology to treat disease and improve the quality of human lives and the scientific challenges involved in making that potential a reality.

The challenges of technology transfer are considered in Part 3, with chapters examining the nature of relationships between universities, where many scientific discoveries are made, and industry, where they are applied; the government's role in fostering cooperation between academia and industry; the need to balance the conflicting yet legitimate interests of all parties in university-industry collaborations; and the complex relationship between intellectual property rights and technology transfer.

In Part 4 contributors with a wide range of viewpoints explore the difficult and complex issues of ethics, behavior, and values both within science and in society as a whole. Focusing first on the professional values held and expressed by individual scientists, the discussion shifts to an analysis of how scientific misconduct is defined and investigated. An eminent scientist and an ethicist trade viewpoints on the social impact of biotechnology. The section concludes with a critique of the scientific culture and an examination of how certain assumptions (including the notions that science is objective and that technological advance is synonymous with progress) have served to exclude women's health issues from scientific research.

The three chapters in the final section of the book examine the role of government in the development of biotechnology internationally as well as here in the United States. A comparison of American, European, and Japanese approaches to the regulation of drugs is followed by an exposition of the Clinton administration's position on scientific research and the commercialization of biotechnology. The concluding chapter focuses on the federal regulatory process, with an analysis of how the U.S. Environmental Protection Agency develops and refines environmental regulations.

As Julian Huxley, Rice University's first professor of biology, noted in

1924, humanity is always mistrustful of radical change in fields such as biology that touch people's feelings and instincts. Biotechnology presents society with both tremendous opportunities and enormous challenges. It is up to all of us—scientists, health care professionals, attorneys, engineers, and concerned lay people—to respond to these opportunities and challenges. We hope that this volume will both contribute to and encourage broad participation in an important dialogue that will shape the direction of biotechnology in the twenty-first century.

> Larry V. McIntire
> Frederick B. Rudolph
> Institute of Biosciences and Bioengineering
> Rice University

Acknowledgments

T he Institute of Biosciences and Bioengineering at Rice University gratefully acknowledges the generous support of Mr. and Mrs. C. M. Hudspeth of Houston, without which this book would not have been possible. In 1991 the Hudspeths created an endowment fund to establish a series of conferences known as the DeLange Conferences, in memory of Mrs. Hudspeth's parents, Albert and Demaris DeLange. The Second DeLange Conference, *Biotechnology: Science, Engineering, and Ethical Challenges for the Twenty-first Century*, on which this book is based, was held at Rice University, Houston, from February 28 to March 2, 1994.

The Institute also acknowledges the important contributions made to both the conference and this book by Diana Welch, Judith Dickson, Eleanor Mayfield, Janelle Scott, Patricia Gibbons, and the following members of the DeLange Conference Planning Committee: David Hellums, Kathleen S. Matthews, Phillip Bedient, George Schroepfer, Baruch Brody, and Norman Hackerman.

Contents

Part 1

BASIC RESEARCH:
THE FOUNDATION OF BIOTECHNOLOGY

Biotechnology has so suddenly been thrust to the center of public consciousness that the casual observer could be forgiven for thinking that this technology had been developed overnight. This is, of course, not the case.

In a sense, the set of knowledge and techniques now collectively known as biotechnology had its beginnings more than 100 years ago with the discovery of the cellular molecule deoxyribonucleic acid (DNA). But almost a century passed before scientists discovered that DNA is the genetic material that transmits the characteristics of an organism from one generation to the next. In 1953, Francis Crick and James Watson elucidated the structure and function of DNA.

Beginning in about 1970, the pace of innovation increased exponentially; all of the scientific breakthroughs and applications associated with modern biotechnology have occurred in the past 25 to 30 years. However, this revolution would not have been possible without the body of basic scientific knowledge that had accumulated before that time.

Like most technological advances, biotechnology has its roots in scientific curiosity: the desire to better understand the biological basis of human life. The importance of basic scientific research—research aimed solely at increasing knowledge—is a theme that runs through these first chapters. In the words of Anna Marie Skalka, of the Fox Chase Cancer Center's Institute for Cancer Research and author of Chapter 2, "research designed simply to answer general problems posed by nature often yields the most far-reaching rewards."

This point is reinforced by Alexander Wlodawer of the National Cancer Institute, author of Chapter 3, who notes that basic research conducted years ago on "obscure chicken viruses" is the foundation for almost everything modern science knows about the human immunodeficiency virus (HIV) that causes acquired immune deficiency syndrome (AIDS).

In Chapter 1, Kathleen Matthews of Rice University describes the nature of the genetic material DNA and indicates how basic research studies on bacteria led to the discovery of restriction enzymes that recognize specific DNA sequences and act as molecular scissors. These proteins make it possible to generate reproducible sets of DNA fragments and led quickly to the ability to separate and analyze DNA, to combine DNA from different organisms, to amplify or clone DNA, and to map genes.

Recombinant DNA technology makes possible the use of living cells as factories for the production of proteins (the basis of the biotechnology industry) as well as the development of transgenic plants and animals (which contain genes transplanted from other species). The ability to fragment and analyze DNA has led to the Human Genome Project, an international effort to map the entire human genome.

Skalka and Wlodawer describe ways in which DNA analysis and recombination technologies are being used to advance understanding and treatment of two of the most complex, mystifying diseases of the modern era: AIDS and cancer. Although these two chapters are probably the most difficult in the book for nonscientists, they offer a glimpse at the frontiers of current research, where answers are being sought to basic questions about cell and molecular biology.

In the final chapter of Part 1, C. Thomas Caskey of Baylor College of Medicine discusses the implications of biotechnology for the diagnosis, treatment, and prevention of disease, raising some of the ethical questions that will be addressed in greater depth later in the book.

1

Overview of Terminology and Advances in Biotechnology

KATHLEEN S. MATTHEWS

Over the past 50 years, the face of biological science has been transformed by discoveries that began at midcentury with the identification of genetic material. The pace of discovery has increased significantly in the past two decades with our ability to manipulate and examine genetic material. The barriers between subdisciplines within the biological sciences have been eroded, and we can now speak of common tools and insights that transcend disciplinary boundaries.

Genetic material is the information that is passed from generation to generation within organisms. These stored and then transmitted data determine all of the activities carried out within a living organism. Genetic information is required for development, differentiation of cells, maintenance of cell function, and reproduction, not just of each cell within an organism, but for the organism itself. Because changes in this genetic material will be passed to subsequent generations, an alteration that affects function will also be passed from one generation to the next.

DNA IDENTIFIED AS GENETIC MATERIAL

Deoxyribonucleic acid (DNA) was known to exist in cells long before it was identified as the genetic material. It was named on the basis of its properties: it contains the sugar ribose missing an oxygen at a specific position (deoxyribose), it is located in the nucleus (nucleic), and it has the properties of an acid. DNA was not identified as genetic material until almost 100 years after its discovery in the cell.

3

Avery et al. (1944) were the first to demonstrate that this material actually contained information that was passed from generation to generation. They accomplished this feat by using two different strains of *Pneumococcus* bacteria. The first strain caused pneumonia and death when injected into mice. In contrast, the second, a very closely related strain, did not cause disease when injected into mice. After fractionating the pathogenic bacterial strain into the different components that are found in cells (protein, DNA, lipids, etc.) and mixing these components individually with the nonpathogenic strain, Avery and colleagues monitored for an ability to transform the bacteria from nonpathogenic to pathogenic. They found that *only* DNA could accomplish this transformation. In addition, the bacteria that were transformed were permanently transformed: not only had the genetic material been altered, but this alteration was passed to subsequent generations. This experiment provided the first direct demonstration that DNA could serve as genetic material.

COMPOSITION OF DNA

DNA is composed of four different components called "bases." These are assembled into structures like beads on a string. The bases have the chemical composition and chemical structure shown in Figure 1-1; these components are linked together in various sequences in different DNAs through the sugar moiety and phosphate to form a deoxyribose-phosphate backbone that forms a scaffold for the bases. In DNA, two single strands come together and form a double-helical structure in which the individual strands run in opposite directions; that is, their relative orientation is antiparallel. The connections to form the sugar-phosphate backbone within each strand are covalent (strong interactions that are difficult

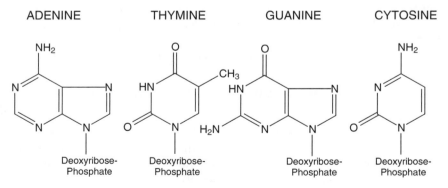

FIGURE 1-1 Components of DNA.

to break), whereas base pairing interactions are weaker (noncovalent bonds) and occur between bases on different strands. The latter interactions stabilize the double-stranded structure of DNA. The individual DNA strands can be separated by changing conditions (e.g., stressing the molecule by increasing temperature), a property that can be useful experimentally.

Another property of DNA is that the four bases, thymine (T), adenine (A), cytosine (C), and guanine (G), are able to form only certain base pairs. T and A always pair, and C and G always pair. Given the antiparallel arrangement of two strands in DNA, if the sequence of one strand is known, the sequence of the other strand can be deduced from these base-pairing rules. The diameter of the DNA molecule is constant regardless of the molecule's length. The length of the bacterial genome is on the order of millions of base pairs; in humans, the length of the DNA chain is about 30 billion base pairs.

DNA SEQUENCE ENCODES PROTEINS

Genetic information is stored in the *sequence* of the base pairs within the DNA (Figure 1-2). This information is copied, or transcribed, into an intermediary message that is used as a template for the assembly of amino acids into the class of molecules called proteins. Proteins are composed of 20 different amino acids that are also assembled somewhat like beads on a string. Three bases in DNA—and consequently in the messenger ribonucleic acid (RNA) intermediary—are used to specify an amino acid. The adjacent triplet of bases specifies a different amino acid and so on throughout the entire sequence of the protein. This translation process alone, however, is not sufficient to generate a functional species.

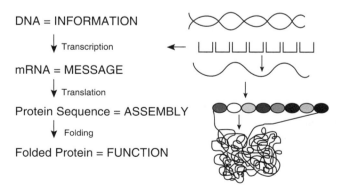

DNA = INFORMATION

↓ Transcription

mRNA = MESSAGE

↓ Translation

Protein Sequence = ASSEMBLY

↓ Folding

Folded Protein = FUNCTION

FIGURE 1-2 DNA makes RNA makes protein.

Each of the amino acids contains a side chain that confers specific chemical properties such that specific interactions can form between amino acids. Amino acids in a particular sequence are able to fold into a specific three-dimensional structure that gives rise to function. In this way, the information that is contained in DNA is converted to functional form. Because the sequence of amino acids varies according to DNA sequence, proteins come in a variety of sequences, shapes, and sizes. Most importantly, proteins are able to perform a variety of functions based on their size and shape.

Protein molecules carry out the myriad of functions characteristic of living organisms. For example, enzymes are proteins that catalyze metabolic reactions in cells. Other proteins serve structural roles; others control differentiation, development, and growth; still others are used in defense. Proteins are the functional expression of genetic material.

MUTATIONS

A gene is the segment of DNA that encodes a protein (or polypeptide). A gene is basically a blueprint for the construction of a protein sequence. Any change in DNA sequence is called a mutation. A mutation can be as small as a single base pair change or it can be an insertion or a deletion or inversion of segments of the sequence. A change in the DNA changes the mRNA and consequently the protein that is assembled from this sequence. When a different amino acid or set of amino acids is incorporated into the protein product, folding into a functional structure may be altered. A mutation can result in an incompletely folded and therefore nonfunctional protein or a protein that is folded in a way that diminishes function.

Mutations can have positive effects, although what are usually observed are negative effects on proteins that result in some deleterious effect on the organism. Perhaps one of the most illustrative examples is the mutation that results in sickle cell anemia. A single base pair change alters the gene that codes for one of the two chains in hemoglobin, the oxygen carrier in red blood cells. This change results in the alteration of the properties of the intact hemoglobin molecule such that the molecules now aggregate within the cell. This aggregation alters the shape of the cell from its normal jelly donut shape, which moves easily through the capillaries, into a sickle shape, hence the name of the disease. When this change happens, the capillaries are occluded, and the cells in blood cannot circulate effectively. As a consequence, oxygen concentration in the blood drops, an event that further promotes hemoglobin aggregation, and the person enters a sickle cell crisis. All of these effects result from a single change in the DNA sequence.

Genes must be identified within the DNA for the transcription process to occur. There are controlling sequences and signaling sequences that indicate the start of a gene and which strand should be copied in which direction. Furthermore, there are regulatory sequences that determine when, how much, and under what conditions a particular protein is produced. It is the constellation of proteins produced over time and within the different types of cells in an organism that determines developmental processes, controls cell differentiation, maintains cell type, etc.

FRAGMENTATION OF DNA

The fact that DNA is a very long and skinny molecule complicated its chemical and physical analysis for many years after its structure was known. By analogy, managing a detailed study of a train that stretches from here to the sun (comparable length:diameter relationship for human DNA) would be simpler if it were possible to fragment the train reproducibly into smaller and more manageable pieces. Until the mid-1970s, there was very little hope of doing that with DNA because the methods available were not very successful and, of utmost importance, were not very reproducible. Out of basic research studies on bacteria came the discovery of a family of enzymes, called restriction nucleases, that can recognize a specific sequence of bases in DNA and act as molecular scissors. The importance of this discovery was that for any given DNA the products were consistently the same. It was therefore possible to generate a *reproducible* set of fragments every time a particular DNA was treated with a particular restriction enzyme. There are now several hundred different restriction enzymes in our arsenal that recognize different sequences reproducibly.

SEPARATION OF DNA AND ANALYSIS

It is equally important to be able to separate the pieces of DNA generated by fragmentation. The technique of electrophoresis provides the opportunity for such separation (Figure 1-3). Mixtures of DNA fragments

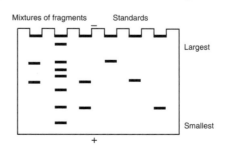

FIGURE 1-3 Separation of DNA fragments.

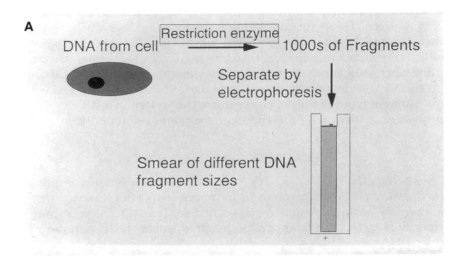

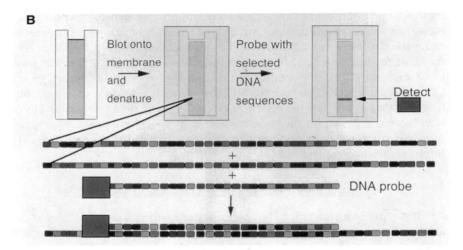

FIGURE 1-4 Restriction fragment length polymorphism (RFLP) analysis (A), probing (B), patterns (C), and applications (D).

can be loaded onto thin gels and subjected to an electric field. Because the charge-to-mass ratio of DNA is independent of fragment length, the largest fragments do not move very far, whereas the smallest fragments move very rapidly through the gel. Standards can be used to identify the size of the DNA fragments, and parts of the gel can be removed to isolate a specific DNA fragment.

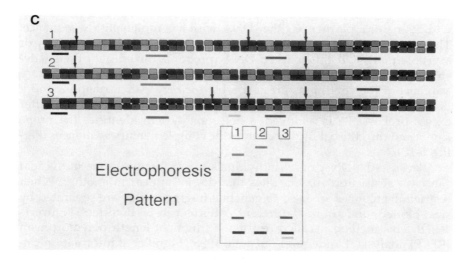

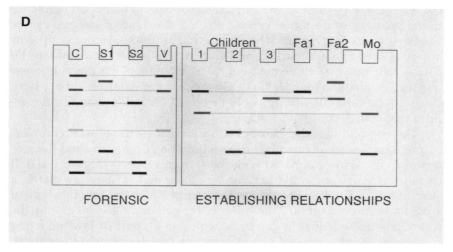

DNA from a human cell can be treated with a restriction enzyme or a set of restriction enzymes to produce thousands of fragments. These can be separated by size via electrophoresis to generate a smear of DNA fragments (Figure 1-4A). If the gel in which this smear is found is blotted onto a support membrane, the DNA will stick to the membrane as the same smear of many individual bands. The membrane can then be treated under conditions that separate the two strands of DNA from one another (Figure 1-4B).

A DNA strand does not discriminate as to whether it is interacting with its natural partner or other DNA with a complementary sequence. Thus, it is possible to take another DNA and mark it with radioactivity or a visible marker. If this marked DNA (probe) is mixed with the single-stranded DNA on the membrane, it will interact with any complementary sequence if the conditions are favorable for base pair formation, and a double-stranded hybrid structure will be generated (Figure 1-4B). After excess probe DNA is removed, a detection system identifies the probe signal and thus the bands that contain the complementary sequences (Figure 1-4B).

Because the DNA of all individuals is not identical, one individual can have restriction enzyme sites that do not appear in another. When restriction enzymes are used to generate fragments that are separated by size, blotted, and probed, different patterns can be detected (Figure 1-4C,D). This method is called restriction fragment length polymorphism (RFLP) analysis (Lander and Botstein, 1986). Significant information can be derived from differences (polymorphisms) in the lengths of restriction fragments. If, for example, the appearance of a particular band correlates to the presence of a specific genetic disease, this type of analysis can be used to identify individuals who have a genetic disease before symptoms appear. Given enough markers and sufficient information about the statistical distribution of those markers in the population, it is possible to use this methodology to identify uniquely an individual (Jeffreys et al., 1986, 1990). In the future it will probably be our DNA rather than our fingerprint that is used for identification.

This method can also be applied in forensic settings where, for example, samples are obtained from a victim or a crime scene and the patterns produced are compared with those from suspects (Figure 1-4D). If there is no match, an individual can be exonerated; if there is a match, a suspect can be implicated in a specific crime. Rules for how this type of analysis is to be done are now becoming generally accepted, and the conditions under which it can be accepted in a court of law are being considered in many states. DNA information can also be used to establish familial relationships (Figure 1-4D). This approach can determine whether a child is the progeny of a particular father and mother.

Beyond the human applications, this type of analysis can be used to determine whether a bacterium carries specific types of drug resistance. This analysis is much faster than the traditional technique of allowing a bacterium to grow in the presence of different drugs as a means of determining drug resistance. There are numerous examples of the application of RFLP analysis.

A method that allows RFLP analysis to be used more widely resulted from being able to amplify specific sequences of DNA. The method is

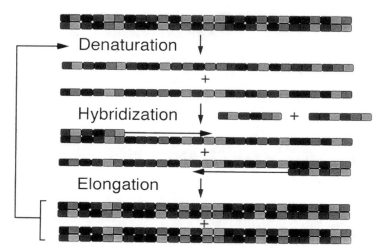

FIGURE 1-5   DNA amplification: polymerase chain reaction (PCR).

called polymerase chain reaction (PCR), and a Nobel Prize was awarded to Kary Mullis for its development (Mullis, 1990). The method is based on the ability to separate the two DNA strands. Because DNA strands are held together by weak forces to form a double-stranded structure, it is possible to separate the two strands. Short sequences of DNA can be made chemically and matched to the ends of each of the strands (Figure 1-5). These short sequences can also form base pairs. By using an enzyme that can recognize this structure and extend, by base pair interactions, each of the short strands, the products are two pieces of DNA that are identical to the original double-stranded DNA. This cycle can be repeated many times to increase the amount of a particular DNA sequence by about a millionfold. Out of a mixture of sequences, a sequence of interest can be uniquely amplified. This amplification allows RFLP analysis on DNA from extremely small samples.

RECOMBINANT DNA

DNA that has been taken apart at specific sequences can be put back together. A sealing enzyme, called ligase, recognizes a gap in DNA and connects the ends, but the action of this enzyme is *not* sequence specific. DNA from two sources can be recombined into one intact segment (called recombinant DNA; Figure 1-6). Thus, the coding sequence for a particular

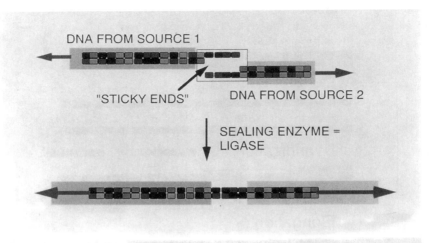

FIGURE 1-6 Connecting different DNAs: Recombinant DNA.

protein can be combined with DNA that belongs to a different organism. This recombinant DNA can be put into the cells of yet another organism for which the product encoded is a foreign protein. Cells of different types can be used as factories for the production of specific proteins. This type of technology forms the basis for the biotechnology industry, producing many types of specific proteins, e.g., hormones, insulin, hemoglobin, tissue plasminogen activator, interleukin, and cytokines.

Obviously, there are important questions about who receives these proteins and under what conditions. There are many issues connected with recombinant DNA technology, and there is even more complicated technology. Not only can a foreign gene be put into the cells of an organism: the gene can actually be incorporated into the DNA derived from germ cells or embryonic cells of another organism. From this combination, an embryo can be produced that contains this gene that came originally from another species (called a transgene). Transgenic embryos can be put into an adult female (e.g., a mouse), which will then give birth to mice permanently carrying the transgene. Various lines of transgenic mice are being used for numerous research efforts, from studying human diseases to examining the effects of the expression of a particular protein in a specific organ. There are also transgenic cows, sheep, pigs, and plants.

What is forbidden, at the moment, is the production of transgenic humans. The National Institutes of Health (NIH) currently forbids any efforts to alter the germ line in humans. Instead, what is being conducted in humans at this time is somatic gene therapy. The altered cells used are not germ-line reproductive cells. The general purpose of these efforts is to use a properly functioning gene to replace a gene that is defective and not operating properly. A retroviral vector is usually used to introduce the transgene into the DNA of cells isolated from an individual. The transgenic DNA then carries the foreign gene that encodes a functional protein that can carry out the specific functions missing in the individual. The cells that are put back into the individual generally home to their organ type (e.g., muscle or blood cells), and the needed protein can then be produced in the recipient. The first such trials were on children with a deficiency in adenine deaminase (ADA), which is required for immune function. The disease produced by ADA absence is called severe combined immune deficiency disease, and children with this disease cannot be exposed to the environment because their immune systems are not functioning. NIH has carried out trials in which the ADA gene was introduced into the cells isolated from an individual, and these cells were then reintroduced into the body. The needed protein was produced in amounts sufficient to allow the treated children to be out in the environment and to assume more normal lives. Now there are at least tens and no doubt soon to be hundreds of different trials for different kinds of gene therapy in attempts to correct a specific genetic deficiency.

SEARCHING FOR SPECIFIC GENES

Gene identification, that is, identifying the coding regions for proteins that have particular functions, is one major purpose for mapping the human genome. A genetic map charts a sequence of characteristics that we know are derived from a particular segment of DNA (Figure 1-7). The Human Genome Project is concerned with putting all human genetic and physical information together in an integrated map. Sequences are also being determined for DNA from other organisms: mice; fruit flies (*Drosophila*); worms (*Caenorhabditis*), where we know a lot about differentiation and development; plants (*Arabidopsis* is a good example); bacteria; yeast; and various others. One surprise is that there is a lot of similarity between mice and humans. What distinguishes humans from mice is much less extensive than might be expected, given the morphology and the characteristics that we associate with these organisms. The commonality as well as the differences in sequence will give us information about living organisms, their development, and the mechanisms that generate the diversity inherent in the living world.

- # Physical Map
  Places selected
  sequences (*e.g.*, cities)

- # Genetic Map
  Places characteristics
  (*e.g.*, Grand Canyon)

- # Sequence
  Puts together all
  information

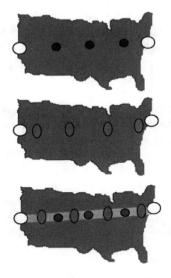

FIGURE 1-7 Mapping the genome.

REFERENCES

Avery, O. T., C. M. MacLeod, and M. McCarty. 1944. Studies on the chemical nature of the substance inducing transformation of pneumococcal types. Inductions of transformation by a deoxyribonucleic acid fraction isolated from pneumococcus type III. J. Exp. Med. 79:137-158.

Jeffreys, A. J., V. Wilson, S. L. Thein, D. J. Wetherall, and B. A. Ponder. 1986. DNA "fingerprints" and segregation analysis of multiple markers in human pedigrees. Am. J. Hum. Genet. 39:11-24.

Jeffreys, A. J., M. Turner, and P. Debenham. 1990. The efficiency of multilocus DNA fingerprint probes for individualization and establishment of family relationships, determined from extensive casework. Am. J. Hum. Genet. 48:824-840.

Lander, E. S., and D. Botstein. 1986. Strategies for studying heterogeneous genetic traits in humans by using a linkage map of restriction fragment length polymorphism. Proc. Natl. Acad. Sci. 83:7353-7357.

Mullis, K. B. 1990. The unusual origin of the polymerase chain reaction. Sci. Amer. April: 56.

2

Advances in Cell and Molecular Biology

ANNA MARIE SKALKA

The era of molecular biology traces its origin to the study of micro-organisms, tiny bacteria and the still smaller viruses, which had aroused the interest of a small group of born-again physicists. This group of scientists was interested in such microorganisms because of their relative simplicity, which seemed to offer the potential for understanding the physical basis of heredity and an answer to the question, What is life?

The work of these molecular biology pioneers was enormously successful. It led to the revelation that the blueprint for clearly inherited genetic traits and for the biochemical functions common to all living cells is encoded in DNA. The efforts of these early molecular biologists also helped to delineate the major metabolic pathways that all cells use to maintain and reproduce themselves. Finally, the knowledge gained from these studies of simple microorganisms also produced the major tools of today's biotechnology industry: bacteria that serve as factories for the production of virtually any desired protein and viruses or plasmid DNAs that serve as vehicles for amplification of any desired gene.

The reason for the success of their efforts is illustrated in Table 2-1, which contains a comparison of the approximate genetic content of these microorganisms and other more complex organisms, as well as information concerning their reproduction potential. The enormous range in the amount of genetic material is apparent from estimates of genome sizes. The early molecular biologists believed that they had a hope of understanding a genome of 45 thousand or even 4 or 10 million base pairs, but there seemed to be no chance of coming to grips with genomes of higher

15

TABLE 2-1   Genome Size and Reproductive Potential[a]

	Genome Size (base pairs in thousands)	Progeny Yield per Gestation Period
Viruses (bacteriophage λ)	45	100/30 minutes
Bacteria (*E. coli*)	4,000	2/20 minutes
Yeast (baker's)	10,000	2/120 minutes
Fruit Fly	180,000 (×2)	~10/24 hours
Mouse	23,000,000 (×2)	~10/3 weeks
Human	28,000,000 (×2)	~1/9 months

[a]Source for genome sizes: Lewin, 1974.

organisms, which were orders of magnitude larger in size. The other advantage of microorganisms is their rapid reproduction rate; for example, yields of approximately 100 viruses from one infected bacterium in 30 minutes or a doubling of bacterial or yeast cells every 20 minutes to 2 hours. Thus, it would be possible to analyze the effects of genetic changes in such organisms in a matter of hours or days. The gestation periods of higher organisms, however, are measured in hours, weeks, and months. It is clear from this comparison why the fast-reproducing fruit fly was a favored model of early genetics for studying multicellular organisms.

Despite the extraordinary success of these early studies, there are certain fundamental questions that these experiments could not address. The living, single-cell microorganisms that were used as models do not face the problems of community living that exist for the cells of multicellular, complex organisms such as humans, mice, or fruitflies. The profoundly different cells that make up the tissues and organs of our bodies all come from a single fertilized egg. They reach their final form and number through a complex series of tightly regulated proliferation cycles and morphological changes. We now know that these changes are a response to signaling between individual cells and between cells and their environment. The details of these processes of cellular differentiation and embryonic development are still largely obscure. These are the mysteries that we are now just beginning to unravel in the modern era of cell and molecular biology.

THE GENETIC REVOLUTION

It is difficult to discuss the expansion in our knowledge of biological processes without acknowledging the technological advances that have made such progress possible. Scientific discovery and technology are inextricably connected. Methods are often created to address specific scientific questions, and the use of novel techniques invariably uncovers new biological phenomena. The unique advantages afforded by modern scientific technological breakthroughs are nowhere more apparent than in the enormous increase in our capacity to perform sophisticated genetic and molecular analyses in higher organisms. Heralded as the genetic revolution, application of new techniques for gene mapping, isolation, and sequencing is fueling efforts to identify and understand the genetic components of human disease. Announcements in the literature, or even in the press, of some new, important discovery occur almost daily.

Our increased ability to manipulate genomes—to introduce extra genes or to modify existing genes in chromosomes—has made it possible to investigate gene function not only at the level of an isolated cell, but also in the context of the whole organism. Thus, we can now look forward to understanding the genetic and biochemical basis of normal embryonic development and cellular differentiation with the same success as the early molecular biologists elucidated the genetic determinants of pathways of metabolism in single-celled microorganisms. We can also hope to understand the molecular basis of defects in these processes caused by genetic lesions, environmental insults, or infectious agents. Medical sciences have already begun to use this knowledge for diagnosing, treating, and preventing disease; for improving the environment; and in agriculture. Examples are numerous. Because my scientific expertise is in the areas of cancer and virology, I will use a few examples from these disciplines to illustrate the current state of our knowledge and the range of challenges and opportunities that seem to be on the horizon.

CANCER (A GENETIC DISEASE)

One of the most important contributions of the modern era of molecular biology is an understanding of the genetic basis of cancer. The fact that cancer incidence rises dramatically with age suggested to epidemiologists some time ago that cancer may be caused by an accumulation of genetic insults (estimated at three to seven; Vogelstein and Kinzler, 1993) over an individual's lifetime. We now know that cancer does arise from succeeding populations of cells in which more and more of these mutations have accumulated. We also know that the critical mutations are those that interfere at various steps in the pathways that regulate intracellular communication, proliferation, and differentiation. The result is uncontrolled cell growth, increasing disorganization, and, finally, malignancy.

A well-documented example of genes altered in colon cancer, uncovered through analysis of tissues isolated from different stages in the gradual evolution of tumors of the colon, is summarized in Figure 2-1. Genes that are the sites of the most frequent mutations observed in colon

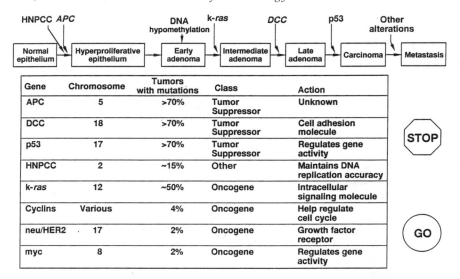

Gene	Chromosome	Tumors with mutations	Class	Action
APC	5	>70%	Tumor Suppressor	Unknown
DCC	18	>70%	Tumor Suppressor	Cell adhesion molecule
p53	17	>70%	Tumor Suppressor	Regulates gene activity
HNPCC	2	~15%	Other	Maintains DNA replication accuracy
k-ras	12	~50%	Oncogene	Intracellular signaling molecule
Cyclins	Various	4%	Oncogene	Help regulate cell cycle
neu/HER2	17	2%	Oncogene	Growth factor receptor
myc	8	2%	Oncogene	Regulates gene activity

FIGURE 2-1   Genes altered in colon cancers. Source: Vogelstein and Kinzler (1993).

cancer and the stages at which they seem to be most critical are shown at the top of the figure. They include two genes known to be involved in two types of familial colon cancer, HNPCC (hereditary nonpolyposis colon cancer) and APC (adenomatus polyposis *coli*), and others including the *ras*, DCC (deleted in colon cancer), and p53 genes. Also included in Figure 2-1 are some less frequently observed mutations, including mutations in oncogenes and tumor suppressor genes. Oncogene mutations cause dominant, gain-of-function changes. By dominant we mean that only one of the pair of genes that we inherit from our father and mother need be affected to trigger the process of uncontrolled cell growth; the mutant gene function overrides that of the normal gene. Because tumor suppressor genes are negative regulators of cell proliferation, both genes must be damaged to cause a release of the critical brake they impose on tumor growth. One analogy for describing the effects of these two types of mutations is an automobile with two sets of controls, the kind used to teach new drivers. There are two ways in which such an automobile might speed out of control. One would be if one of the gas pedals got stuck. If this happened, it would not matter that the second pedal (or normal gene) functioned appropriately; the car would still be out of control. The gas pedal problem would be analogous to an oncogene mutation. However, if the car were out of control because one of the brake pedals did not function, it could still be stopped with the second brake pedal. Thus, as with the tumor suppressor genes, for all braking function to be lost, both brake pedals must fail. Both types of mutations, but more frequently mutations in one copy of a tumor suppressor gene, can occur in our germ cells and be passed on to our descendants. These lead to inborn, heritable predispositions to cancer. One brake is already gone and a second hit on the other will be disastrous. Although such inherited cancers are relatively rare, study of their genetic components has provided great insight into the etiology of the more common sporadic, or acquired, cancers because the very same genetic players are ultimately involved.

At first, the list in Figure 2-1 seems daunting and helps to explain why the war on cancer has been waging so long. We do know that at least in some cases, when a single, normal tumor suppressor gene is provided to a cancer cell with numerous mutations, proliferation and invasive properties can be inhibited dramatically. Therefore, the multiple players may, in fact, provide multiple targets for intervention. In any case, information of the sort provided by studies such as these has already proved useful for diagnosis, for determining prognosis, and in managing the care of cancer patients.

Some of these mutations, for example, those involving gene p53, are common to many malignancies. They are currently the focus of intense study. The HNPCC defect is estimated to occur in one of every 200 individuals in the population (Lynch et al., 1993). Affected individuals can develop tumors of the colon, uterus, ovary, and other organs. The responsible gene (hMSH2), whose identity and function were discovered recently, is required to repair copying mistakes in DNA replication (Fishel et al., 1993; Kinzler et al., 1993; Leach et al., 1993; Parsons et al., 1993). In its normal role this gene can be thought of as a text editor. The loss of its function shows up as an accumulation of mistakes (mutations at many sites in the genome), some of which are oncogenic. Efforts are already underway to develop screening tests for this mutation to use for members of families in which colon cancer is prevalent. Presumably individuals found to carry a mutant form of this gene would then undergo routine periodic testing so that malignancies could be detected at the earliest stage, when treatment would be most effective.

What about treatment? How can modern cell and molecular biology make a contribution in this area? On the basis of types of action deduced for the genes involved in cancer, two types of treatments may be envisioned. One, a seemingly rational approach for compensating for the loss of tumor suppressor gene function, would be to replace the gene. The other, for oncogenes where mutations trigger aberrant function, would be to counter malfunction. Developing such strategies will require a comprehensive understanding of the mechanism of action and the roles of the normal counterparts of these genes in the molecular biology of the cell.

There are some promising starts, for example, the progress in our understanding of the function of the protein that is encoded by *ras*; *ras* is one of the most commonly detected oncogenes in human tumors and has been studied by many workers for more than a decade. Figure 2-2 shows a simplified illustration of the type of signaling pathways maintained by the cells of higher organisms that allow them to judge the status of their neighbors, to ensure proper attachments to tissue contact points, and to respond to the presence of growth factors, hormones, and other external signals. The pathway consists of chains of communicating proteins that receive signals from upstream (starting at the surface of the cell) and pass them to downstream targets known as effectors. The process is complex and includes chemical changes that are catalyzed after direct contact of the protein members. Furthermore, most (or all) of the proteins in the pathway can interact with multiple effectors. The Ras protein was long known to be a key player in these pathways. Despite this knowledge it is only recently that all of the steps could be put together in a fully connected framework (Egan and Weinberg, 1993).

The Ras protein (coded by *ras* gene) is a universal signal receptor, receiving messages initiated at a number of different cell surface receptors after they are stimulated by specific ligands, such as growth factors.

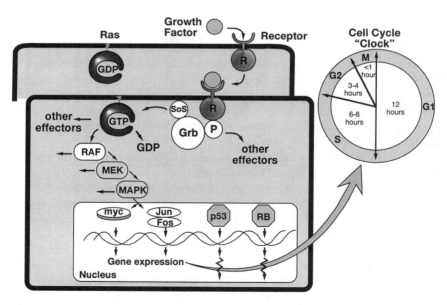

FIGURE 2-2   The *ras* signaling pathway.

The protein comes in two forms; one is silent (no signal is passed) and the other is activated for signal transduction. The protein produced by the mutant *ras* oncogene is activated inappropriately, without having received a signal from an upstream receptor. The Ras protein is anchored in the inner membrane of the cell, ready to make contact with various receptor complexes and to relay the message of this interaction through a cascade of phosphorylating enzymes (kinases) to the nucleus.

Many of the members of the pathway are proteins encoded by previously identified oncogenes (e.g., *raf, myc, jun*), illustrating that defects anywhere along the pathway can have the same ultimate effect. The final targets of this pathway are nuclear transcription factors that respond by turning on the expression of specific genes. In the case of growth factors, genes required for proliferation are turned on. They then start up the cell cycle clock, which leads to DNA replication (the S phase), mitosis (the M phase), and division into two new cells. The proteins encoded by the tumor suppressor genes such as RB and p53 also act in the nucleus, but their roles are to put brakes on the cell cycle by preventing DNA synthesis, allowing repair of DNA damage before cell division, or, when repair cannot be effected, programming the cell to self-destruct.

To receive messages from cell surface receptors, *ras* must be anchored at the inner surface of the cell membrane (Figure 2-3). This anchoring depends on the use of a small 15-carbon molecule called farnesyl, which also has another role in the cell as a precursor in the pathway of cholesterol biosynthesis. Mutational analyses and studies with inhibitors of cholesterol biosynthesis have shown that Ras protein molecules lacking farnesyl do not attach to the cell membrane and cannot participate in signal transduction. The enzyme that performs this attachment, called farnesyltransferase, recognizes and binds the precursor, farnesyl-diphosphate, as well as a short amino acid sequence at the very end of the Ras protein (Figure 2-4). The enzyme then attaches the farnesyl moiety to the Ras protein. This reaction and farnesyltransferase are the target of current approaches to the design of inhibitors of Ras.

The approaches are based on the synthesis of molecules that look like either of the two substrates and will bind to the active site of the enzyme, thus interfering with attachment (Gibbs, 1991). Recent results from several laboratories look very encouraging (Kohl et al., 1993; James et al., 1993). These new inhibitors appear to interfere dramatically with the growth of tissue culture cells that express the activated form of Ras and proliferate in multilayered clumps that mimic cancerous growth. Most encouraging is the relative lack of toxicity of these inhibitors for normal cells or cells that are cancerous because of the expression of some other oncogene. Although much more needs to be done before such drugs can be used to treat people, it now seems increasing possible that inhibitors of

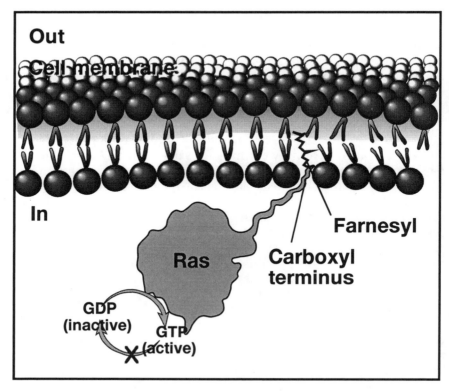

FIGURE 2-3 Ras anchoring at the inner surface of the cell membrane. Source: Touchette (1990).

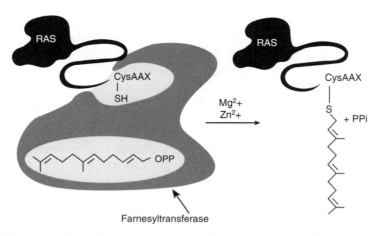

FIGURE 2-4 Action of farnesyltransferase. Source: Tamanoi (1993).

TABLE 2-2   Diseases Targeted by Gene Therapies:
Affected Populations (United States)

Disease/Condition	Incidence (annual)
Cancers	
Brain Tumors[a]	16,700
Breast Cancer[a]	175,000
Colon Cancer[a]	157,500
Leukemia[a]	29,300
Lymphoma[a]	43,000
Melanoma[a]	32,000
Myeloma, Multiple[a]	12,800
Non-small Cell Lung Cancer[a]	100,000
Renal Carcinoma	27,200
Genetic Diseases	
Anemia	50,000-100,000
Cystic Fibrosis[a]	30,000
Gaucher Disease[a]	20,000
Hemophilia (P)[b]	23,000
Hemoglobinopathies	50,000
Hypercholesterolemia[a]	250
Hypopituitary	10,000-15,000
SCID[a](P)	<40
High Cholesterol (P)	60,000,000
Others	
HIV[a]	35,000
Inherited Emphysema	20,000-40,000

[a]In gene therapy trials.
[b]Prevalence.

Sources: American Cancer Society and the Centers for Disease Control and Prevention.

this kind, designed through knowledge of molecular aspects of critical intracellular reactions, will be among the first to emerge as new clinical candidates for anticancer therapy.

Gene therapy is another experimental approach to cancer. As can be seen from Table 2-2, together with the indicated heritable genetic disorders, cancers are a major target for gene therapy protocols in the United States. These treatments attempt to manipulate oncogene or tumor suppressor gene expression in cancer cells to ameliorate or reverse the process. Another strategy for gene therapy is to transfer genes that will stimulate immunity against cancer cells. Many of these approaches to cancer treatment also look promising, although initial attempts have shown that there is still much to be learned about gene delivery systems and the immune system before gene therapy can be considered a straightforward exercise (Miller, 1992).

ACQUIRED IMMUNE DEFICIENCY SYNDROME

Nowhere has our lack of sufficient fundamental knowledge about the body's immune defenses been more apparent than in our confrontation with acquired immune deficiency syndrome (AIDS; caused by the human immunodeficiency virus, HIV), which is another major target for gene therapy. HIV is particularly pernicious because it attacks the cells (called T cells) needed to mount an effective defense against infection. It enters these cells by attaching to a cell surface receptor (called CD4) that is a key component in the cell-to-cell communication that must occur during an immune response. This inappropriate interaction and others that occur after viral entry trigger responses in these cells that adversely affect the immune system both directly and indirectly. Some indirect effects appear to be responsible for damage to the central nervous system, giving rise to AIDS-related dementia. Efforts to develop vaccines have also been stymied because it still not clear what features of an immune response actually confer even transient protection against AIDS. Presumably, the immune system responds to components in the outer coat of the virus. However, HIV can rapidly mutate its genome during replication, allowing it to alter its outer coat. These two properties, direct attack on the immune system and variation in the surface it presents, eventually allow the virus to escape immune recognition entirely. Such problems have further confounded efforts to develop vaccines against AIDS.

The HIV life cycle is quite complex (Figure 2-5). Furthermore, gaps in our understanding of the host cell machinery that the virus takes over and of the nature of the control that the virus exerts on its own gene expression have made it difficult to intervene in the intermediate stages in the viral life cycle. Here and in other aspects of viral pathogenesis, the need for more fundamental knowledge is clear. Although not yet entirely satisfactory, the only approach that has yielded drugs that have been approved in the United States for the treatment of AIDS is targeted against the viral-specific enzymes encoded in the virus genome and essential at very early and very late replication stages (Katz and Skalka, 1994).

The targeted enzymes include the reverse transcriptase that the virus brings with it into the cell that it infects (and uses to convert its genetic information into a chemical form that is compatible with that of the host) and the protease that is required for processing and activating the virus' structural proteins and enzymes. The currently used reverse-transcriptase inhibitors (e.g., AZT, ddI, DDC, and d4T) are all analogs of the building blocks of DNA that interfere with viral DNA synthesis. Design of inhibitors for this enzyme and for the protease (discussed in more detail in this symposium by Dr. Wlodawer) have been aided significantly by the availability of detailed structural information concerning these proteins and

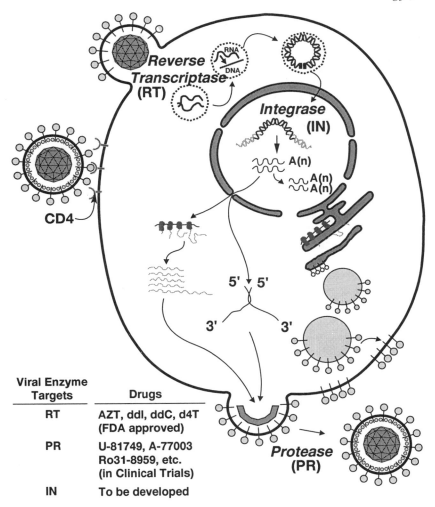

Viral Enzyme Targets	Drugs
RT	AZT, ddl, ddC, d4T (FDA approved)
PR	U-81749, A-77003 Ro31-8959, etc. (in Clinical Trials)
IN	To be developed

FIGURE 2-5 The life cycle of HIV.

their mechanisms of action. Although the challenge of turning structural insights into effective treatments remains formidable, these enzymes offer some of the best models for modern, rational drug design. Studies of the third enzyme, the integrase that the virus uses to splice its DNA into that of the host cell, are not as far along. This enzyme functions at a key step in the viral life cycle, one that allows the infection to persist for the life of the infected cell and all of its daughter cells. Because of its importance, our laboratory and others are striving to obtain more detailed mechanistic and structural information. We have devised simple test tube assays for integrase that can be used to screen for and test inhibitors.

Unfortunately, HIV has already shown that it can mutate rapidly enough to eventually escape treatment with one anti-reverse transcriptase drug. The hope of current efforts is that attack at multiple targets will produce additive or synergistic effects that will eventually halt virus spread, prolong lives, and prevent establishment of infection in people newly exposed to the virus.

SUMMARY

Modern advances in cellular and molecular biology have expanded opportunities and delineated new challenges in biomedical research. However, despite the best of efforts, this glimpse into the future can only be considered limited. Two additional variables will surely be part of the picture but, unfortunately, are impossible to assess.

For predicting scientific advances the missing variable is serendipity. We know that research in one area often produces conceptual breakthroughs and important insights in another, sometimes seemingly unrelated area. Thus, no matter how comprehensive our discussion is today, it is likely—even probable—that we are in for some big surprises from unsuspected directions in the future. If past experience holds true, some of these breakthroughs will have a big practical payoff. Thus, despite the current, public demands for more and more targeted research, we must continue to interpret our biomedical research mandates as broadly as possible. As the history of research into cell and molecular biology illustrates, research designed simply to answer general problems posed by nature often yields the most far-reaching rewards.

For predicting technological advances, the missing variable is improvement in methodologies. Perhaps the most striking example is in the computer industry. The computer currently in use probably was obsolete the day it appeared on the market. Technology, fueled by new knowledge, always seems to get better. With such improvement comes an ever-increasing capacity to explore the myriad of fundamental questions that remain in both cell and molecular biology. With these final thoughts in mind we can look forward to the next new era of cell and molecular biology.

ACKNOWLEDGMENTS

I am grateful to Dr. Allen Oliff of Merck Research Laboratories for discussions and ideas concerning anticancer treatments based on oncogene protein inhibitors; to Dr. Ken Tartof of Fox Chase Cancer Center for providing the table summarizing gene therapy as well as helpful ideas concerning the usefulness of this approach; to my colleague Dr. Richard Katz for constructive suggestions concerning the manuscript; and to Marie Estes for her excellent secretarial assistance. Work in my laboratory is supported by National Institutes of Health grants CA-47486, CA-06927, and RR-05539; a grant from the Pew Charitable Trust; a grant for infectious disease research from Bristol-Myers Squibb Foundation; and an appropriation from the Commonwealth of Pennsylvania. The contents of this manuscript are solely the responsibility of the author and do not necessarily represent the official views of the National Cancer Institute or any other sponsoring organization.

REFERENCES

Egan, S. E., and R. A. Weinberg. 1993. The pathway to signal achievement. Nature 365:781-783.

Fishel, R., M. K. Lescoe, M. R. S. Rao, N. G. Copeland, N. A. Jenkins, J. Garber, M. Kane, and R. Kolodner. 1993. The human mutator gene homolog MSH2 and its association with hereditary nonpolyposis colon cancer. Cell 75:1027-1038.

Gibbs, J. B. 1991. R~ C-terminal processing enzymes—new drug targets? Cell 65:1-4.

James, G. L., J. L. Goldstein, M. S. Brown, T. E. Rawson, T. C. Somers, R. S. McDowell, C. W. Crowley, B. K. Lucas, A. D. Levinson, and J. C. Marsters, Jr. 1993. Benzodiazepine peptidomimetics: Potent inhibitors of *ras* farnesylation in animal cells. Science 260:1937-1942.

Katz, R. A., and A. M. Skalka. 1994. The retroviral enzymes. Annu. Rev. Biochem. 63:133-173.

Kinzler, B. Vogelstein, and P. Modrich. 1993. Hypermutability and mismatch repair deficiency in RER+ tumor cells. Cell 75:1227-1236.

Kohl, N. E., S. D. Mosser, S. J. deSolms, E. A. Giuliani, D. L. Pompliano, S. L. Graham, R. L. Smith, E. M. Scolnick, A. Oliff, and J. B. Gibbs. 1993. Selective inhibition of rr-dependent transformation by a farnesyltransferase inhibitor. Science 260:1934-1937.

Leach, F. S., N. C. Nicolaides, N. Papadopoulos, B. Liu, J. Jen, R. Parsons, P. Peltomaki, P. Sistonen, L. A. Aaltonen, M. Nystrom-Lahti, K. Y. Guan, J. Zhang, P. S. Meltzer, J.-W. Yu, F.-T. Kao, D. J. Chen, K. M. Cerosaletti, R. E. K. Fournier, S. Todd, T. Lewis, R. J. Leach, S. L. Naylor, J. Weissenbach, J.-P. Mecklin, H. Jarvinen, G. M. Petersen, S. R. Hamilton, J. Green, J. Jass, P. Watson, H. T. Lynch, J. M. Trent, A. de la Chapelle, K. W. Kinzler, and B. Vogelstein. 1993. Mutations of a *mutS* homolog in hereditary nonpolyposis colorectal cancer. Cell 75:1215-1225.

Lewin, B., ed. 1974. Structure of the chromosome in gene expression. Pp. 1-47 in Vol 2. Eucaryotic Chromosomes. New York: John Wiley & Sons.

Lynch, P. M., R. J. Cavalieri, and C. R. Boland. 1993. Genetics, natural history, tumor spectrum, and pathology of hereditary nonpolyposis colorectal cancer: an updated review. Gastroenterology 104:1535-1549.

Marx, J. 1993. New colon cancer gene discovered. Science 260:751-752.

Miller, A. D. 1992. Human gene therapy comes of age. Nature 357:455-460.

Parsons, R., G. M. Li, M. J. Longely, W.-H. Fang, N. Papadopoulos, J. Jen, A. de la Chapelle, K. W. Kinzler, B. Vogelstein, and P. Modrich. 1993. Hypermutability and mismatch repair defiicency in RER+ tumor cells. Cell 75:1227-1236.

Tamanoi, F. 1993. Inhibitors of *ras* farnesyltransferases. Trends Biochem. Sci. 18:349-353.

Touchette, N. 1990. Cholesterol and cancer studies get a rise out of yeast. J. NIH Res. 2:61.

Vogelstein, B., and K. W. Kinzler. 1993. The multistep nature of cancer. Trends Genet. 9:138-141.

3

Structural Biology as It Applies to Biotechnology

ALEXANDER WLODAWER

S tructural biology is a large field that has a lot to contribute to biotechnology. I am going to discuss two examples of how information gained by structural biology techniques can be used in structure-based drug design to illustrate the potential of the field. One example has already led to drugs in clinical trials; the other has not led to any drugs as yet and shows how difficult it is to design drugs on the basis of structural data.

Many scientists still say that there is not a truly designed drug on the market and that every drug results from serendipity and medicinal chemistry, with design taking a secondary role. It is necessary, however, to understand what is meant by "design." For example, design could be interpreted as designing a compound to inhibit a particular protein so that disease X will be cured. Imagine that a scientist uses his computer to create such a compound. It inhibits this protein and the disease is gone. If this is how drug design is interpreted, then of course it is true that nothing has ever been designed that way. What is really meant by drug design can be illustrated by using proteins encoded by human immunodeficiency virus (HIV) as an example.

DESIGN OF ANTI-HIV DRUGS

Retroviruses have a unique way of encoding their proteins as so-called polyproteins, in which a number of different proteins are synthesized as contiguous polypeptide chains (Figure 3-1). This property is very

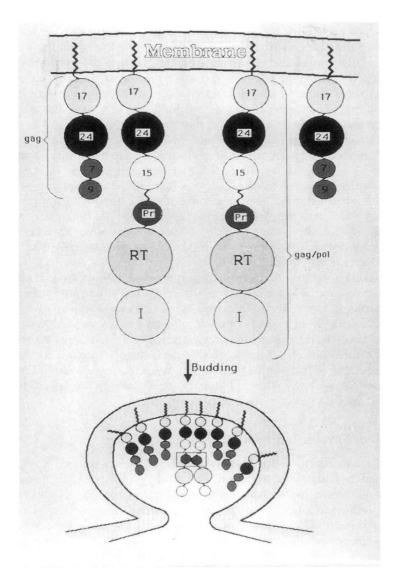

FIGURE 3-1 Schematic diagram of the polyproteins interacting with the cell membrane during budding of human immunodeficiency virus (HIV).

important in the retroviral life cycle, because polyproteins attach themselves to the cell membrane before the budding of viral particles begins; after budding, one of the enzymes encoded by the virus (protease) starts the cascade of cleaving these polyproteins into individual molecules. Exactly how the process starts is still not completely known, but there is no question that protease is responsible for the creation of infectious viral particles. If the enzyme is disabled either by mutation or inhibition, the viral particles that are formed may look normal but are not infectious.

The first structure that was determined was of that of the enzyme without an inhibitor or substrate in its active site (Figure 3-2). The molecule has a very large cavity, and this cavity was suspected of being the site for the catalytic reaction. This enzyme belongs to the family of aspartic proteases. It has two aspartic acids that are in contact, and even before the structure was determined it was speculated that the enzyme would resemble other aspartic proteases, some of which are quite important in humans. One such protease is human renin, which has been a target for drug design for almost two decades. So, a lot was known about how to make inhibitors for this class of proteins even before we knew that HIV would carry one of them.

This is a good time to reiterate the importance of basic research versus targeted research. We would not have been anywhere in the field of retrovirology, as applied to infection by HIV, if many years ago people had not been willing to study obscure chicken viruses. A lot of what we learned about retroviruses came from studies for which utility appeared at that time to be zero. This work was done long before anybody ever heard of acquired immune deficiency syndrome (AIDS), and it is an excellent example of why we should not try to concentrate on the disease of the day and only do targeted research.

Design of Enzyme Inhibitors

How are inhibitors for these types of enzymes designed? First, it is important to understand something about how inhibitors work. Knowing the actual three-dimensional structure may not be completely necessary, but something must be known about the enzymatic properties and function. HIV protease can cleave many different sequences, including all linkages between the proteins in the polyprotein. These sequences can give rise to ideas about designing inhibitors by replacing the peptide bond between the two residues being cleaved by some other chemical group with a structure similar to a peptide bond but resistant to cleavage by the enzyme (Figure 3-3). Again, the choice of all of these inserts is the result of many years of work on the design of inhibitors of human renin

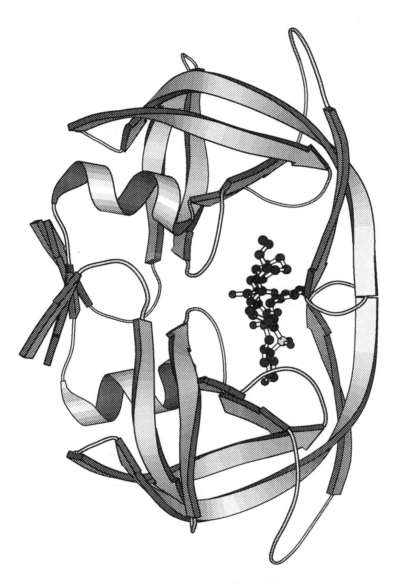

FIGURE 3-2   HIV protease with an inhibitor, PD134922.

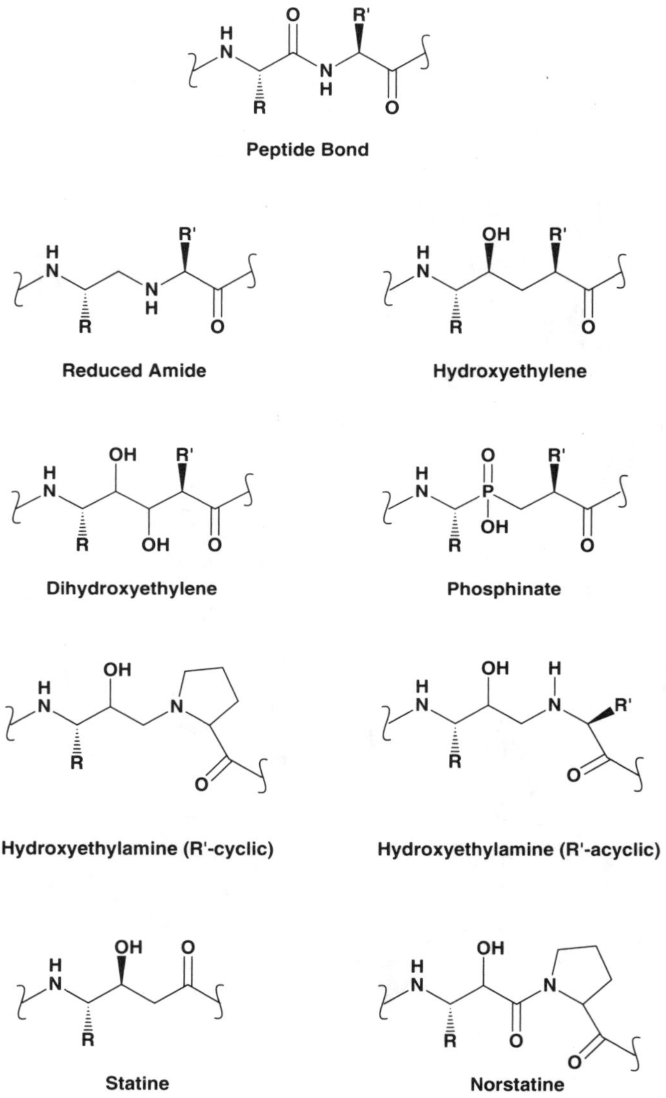

Peptide Bond

Reduced Amide

Hydroxyethylene

Dihydroxyethylene

Phosphinate

Hydroxyethylamine (R'-cyclic)

Hydroxyethylamine (R'-acyclic)

Statine

Norstatine

FIGURE 3-3 Peptide bond and its nonscisssile replacements.

and these data were all in place when scientists started working on HIV protease in the late 1980s.

Many inhibitors of HIV protease have been made, and a selection of them was studied in our laboratory. Some of these compounds are similar to the original substrates; for example, MVT-101 seen in Figure 3-4 uses only standard amino acids. It has the reduced peptide bond in the center and blocking groups at the ends, and that is it. This is a very simple-minded way of producing an inhibitor; other inhibitors contain groups that are not standard amino acids. Peptides usually do not make good drugs because they are susceptible to other proteases present in the organisms, and they do not transport well through membranes. Figure 3-4 is a list of inhibitors studied by crystallography in my laboratory. It is a random list of compounds, not a progression leading to drugs, but all of these structures teach us something about the properties of the target system and the properties of the interactions between the enzyme and the inhibitor.

At least 20 different laboratories have determined at least one structure of HIV protease (Table 3-1), but the number of structures that were actually published and released is rather limited. A very important point emerging from this table is the lack of correlation between the number of structures from a particular laboratory and the number of compounds in clinical trials.

The structure of HIV protease shown previously was that of the apoenzyme. Shown in Figure 3-5 is the structure of an inhibitor complex. What happened in this case was something unexpected. Most enzymes do not change their structure appreciably upon binding of the inhibitors, but some do. In this particular case, there was a large change in the structure: about one-quarter of the molecule showed movements of α-carbon of more than 1 angstrom (0.1 nanometers).

Comparison of Inhibitors

The next step of analysis involves comparing the inhibitors (Figure 3-6, see color plate). Once a series of structures has been created, the structures can be superimposed on one frame and educated guesses about the importance of parts of the molecule can be made. It becomes apparent which parts present in a particular inhibitor are not essential. This is when you can start looking at a number of your different examples and start drawing some overall conclusions from them.

When do you have a number of structures sufficient for beginning analysis? When can you rely on computer analysis and not worry, for example, about crystals or collecting data? Figure 3-7 (see color plate) is an example of a crystal structure of an inhibitor that we determined in

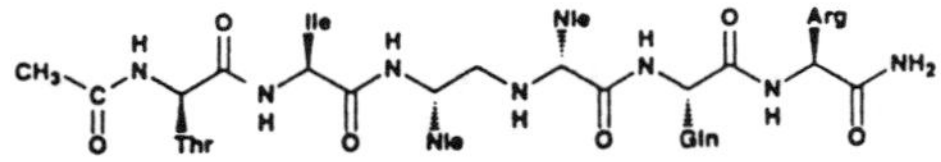

MVT-101
K_I = 780 nM

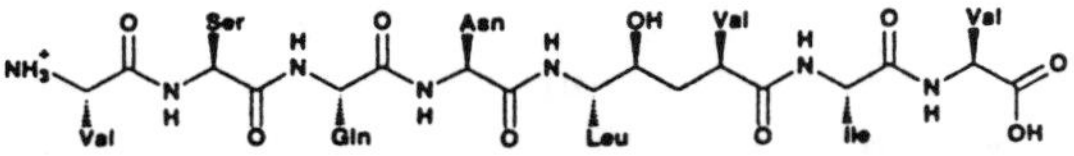

U-85548e
K_I <1 nM

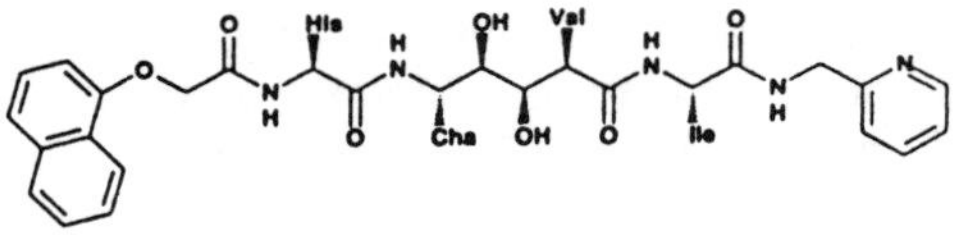

U-75875
K_I = <1.0 nM

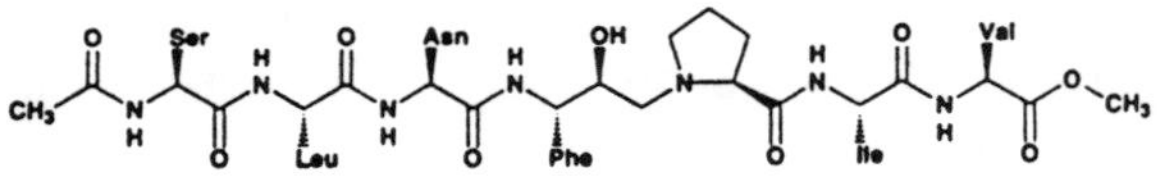

JG-365
K_I = 0.66 nM

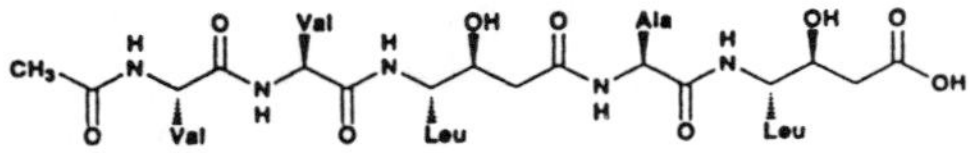

Acetylpepstatin
K_I = 20 nM

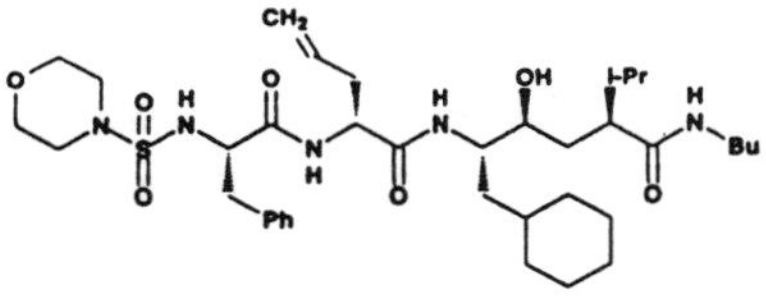

PD-134922
IC_{50} = 15 nM

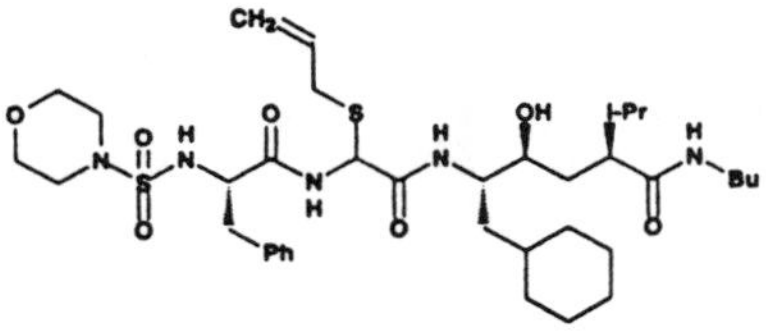

PD-135390
IC_{50} = 2 nM

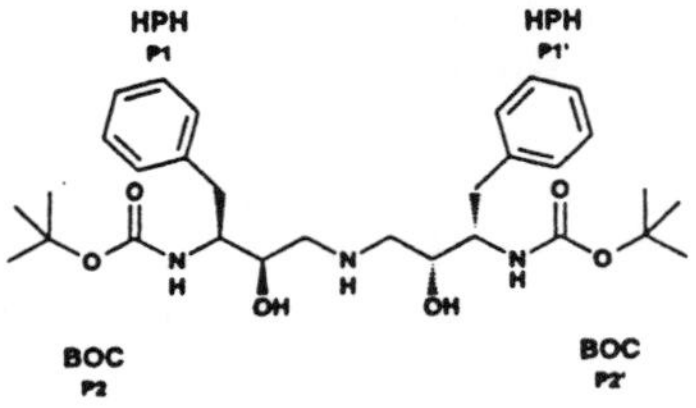

BMS-182193
K_I = 100 nM

FIGURE 3-4 HIV protease inhibitors studied by crystallography in the author's laboratory.

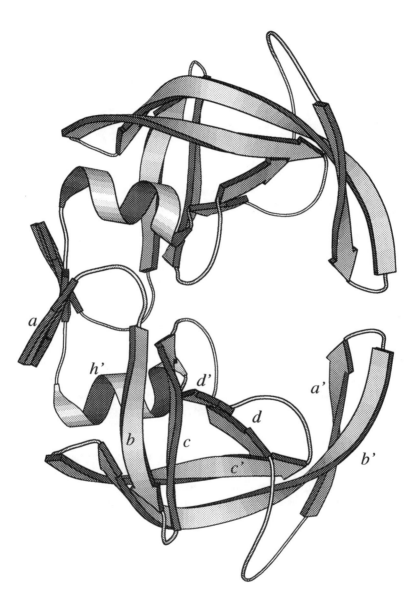

FIGURE 3-5   Native HIV protease.

TABLE 3-1   Studies of Inhibitor Complexes of HIV PR

Laboratory	Location	Structures (No.)	Published (No.)
NCI-ABL	Frederick, Md.	9	5
NCI-PRI	Frederick, Md.	13	5
Merck	Rahway, N.J.	27 (HIV-1), 1 (HIV-2)	7
Abbott	Abbott Park, Ill.	15	1
Roche	Nutley, N.J.	2	2
SmithKline	King of Prussia, Pa.	14 (HIV-1), 2 (SIV)	11
Upjohn	Kalamazoo, Mich.	28 (HIV-1), 28 (HIV-2)	2
Agouron	San Diego, Calif.	50+	8
Dupont-Merck	Wilmington, Del.	36	1
Glaxo	Greenford, England	7	6
UCSF	San Francisco, Calif.	5 (HIV-1), 5 (SIV)	2
Boehringer-Ingelheim	Ridgefield, Conn.	11 (HIV-2)	1
Monsanto	St. Louis, Mo.	22	-
Marion Merrell Dow	Strasbourg, France	8	-
Birkbeck College	London, England	5	-
Ciba	Basel, Switzerland	5	-
Lederle Laboratories	Pearl River, N.Y.	3	-
Eli Lilly	Indianapolis, Ind.	2	-
Oxford/Wellcome	Oxford, England	1	-
Hoechst	Frankfurt, Germany	1	-
Vertex	Cambridge, Mass.	some	-

collaboration with our colleagues from Upjohn who developed the model. Even though many of the features of the model are accurate, examination of the actual hydrogen bonds and the very detailed interactions between the inhibitors and the enzyme shows that the model as a whole is not accurate. Once the structure was determined, the computational chemists were able to recalculate the model with the additional information.

Our predictions of the structure of compounds that will bind to HIV protease are becoming quite good. However, when all experimentally determined structures will be released into public domain, the wealth of experimental structures available will be completely unprecedented. This level of activity has never happened before and is unlikely to happen in the future. We have a chance to learn a lot about how an enzyme works, how the inhibitors work, and about the process of inhibition.

Learning from Design

Have we found anything really unexpected, without which the design of compounds would not be possible or not easy? The answer to this

HIV1 PR – Inh(U85548e)
Water 301

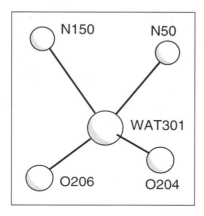

HB Distances (Å)			Angles (°)				
O301	... O204	2.41	O204	... O301	... O206		122
O301	... O206	2.66	O204	... O301	... N50		106
O301	... N50	3.31	O204	... O301	... N150		107
O301	... N150	3.58	O206	... O301	... N50		120
			O206	... O301	... N150		107
			N50	... O301	... N150		91

FIGURE 3-8 HIV1 PR—Inh(U85548e): water 301.

question is yes. What was really unexpected was one water molecule, usually called water-301, that was found in the active site of HIV protease and that is always present in the complex between these specific inhibitors and the protease (Figure 3-8). Analysis of the structure near this particular water molecule reveals that it makes very good hydrogen bonds between two nitrogen atoms belonging to the enzyme and two oxygen atoms belonging to the inhibitor. These interactions were observed in almost all the structures of known inhibitors.

As soon as we saw that there was something very unusual about and very specific to this complex, we and others suggested that it could be useful to try to make compounds that would include an equivalent of this water in the inhibitor itself. That is, of course, easy to postulate but difficult to do. Lam et al. (1994) recently published the structure of such a compound. This inhibitor has a cyclic urea group, where an oxygen atom replaces this particular water. This is one of the first examples of a non-peptidic HIV protease inhibitor that was designed, constructed, and shown to be a very potent antiviral agent. Unfortunately, this compound turned out not to be a good drug. Even though the inhibitor was very highly bioavailable, it was sequestered by the liver, resulting in an unsuccessful clinical trial. Follow-up compounds are being worked on, and there is hope that this approach will ultimately succeed. The problem of whether inhibitors will eventually turn into drugs is very complex, and bioavailability and pharmacokinetics are not easily seen in the structures. The next step involves extensive medicinal chemistry, which is still being done to a large extent by trial and error. That is the story of the HIV protease, which is conceptually a very easy example of drug design, because designing enzyme inhibitors is comparatively simple.

DESIGN OF CYTOKINE AGONISTS AND ANTAGONISTS

Now let us go to something that is not so simple: making agonists and antagonists of cytokines. Understanding cell signaling is one of the most important areas in biology now, because signaling pathways in organisms are elaborate, complicated, and not yet completely understood. The steps in some of these pathways, however, are known.

Knowledge of cytokine structures is relatively recent (Table 3-2). Except for preliminary structures of porcine growth hormone and interleukin 2 (IL-2), only in the past few years have we started seeing this particular class of cytokines in atomic detail. All that we know about the interactions between helical cytokines and their receptors, or actually extracellular parts of the receptors, comes from one publication by de Vos et al. (1992). This publication describes the interactions of human growth hormone with the receptor (Figure 3-9, see color plate). It was an extremely important development, but the choice was unfortunate from the point of view of trying to generalize it for the other systems. It turns out that a single molecule of human growth hormone causes dimerization of two identical molecules of the receptor. Each of the receptors interacts with a completely different part of the cytokine and the receptors use exactly the same part to interact with two different targets. Unfortunately, this is the only known example of these types of interactions, and it has already led us astray trying to understand other cytokines.

TABLE 3-2   Structures of Helical Cytokines

Porcine Growth Hormone	Monsanto	1987
Interleukin 2	Boulder	1987
CM-CSF	Cornell	1991
Interferon γ	UAB, NCI	1991
Human Growth Hormone/Receptor	Genentech	1992
Interleukin 2	Stanford	1992
Interleukin 4	4 structures	1992
Interferon β	Nagaoka	1992
G-CSF	UCLA	1993
M-CSF	Berkeley	1993
Interleukin 5	Glaxo	1993

UAB, University of Alabama at Birmingham; NCI, National Cancer Institute; UCLA, University of California at Los Angeles.

As the structures of cytokines started appearing, we and others noted that they share many similarities. Superposition of IL-2, IL-4, and GM-CSF shows that the core of the protein is very similar although some parts are quite different (Figure 3-10, see color plate). This gives rise to a question of whether the similarity between different cytokines is important and can be used in trying to design cytokine agonists and antagonists. Bazan (1990) showed that regardless of the low or sometimes undetectable similarity among the cytokines themselves, the receptors are very closely related and their extracellular domains have almost the same structure, which is that seen for human growth hormone receptor.

Once we had access to a number of the structures in addition to the amino acid sequences of these cytokines, it was possible to structurally align their sequences. There is a fair amount of similarity, at least in the conserved core, where the superposition is meaningful. In the absence of the structural data, this type of superposition is very difficult; the superpositions of these particular cytokines found in the literature were uniformly wrong.

The parts of the primary and tertiary structure that are most similar include two of the helixes, helix A and helix D (Figure 3-11). Other studies also showed that these particular regions of the cytokines seem to be directly involved in receptor binding, which is why we hope to be able, by modifying these particular areas, to make other molecules that can modify the activities of cytokines.

The interplay between different cytokines and their receptors can get very complicated. The laboratory of Warren Leonard created a picture showing something that became obvious only recently, which has thrown a monkey wrench into this whole field (Figure 3-12, see color plate) (Russell et al., 1993). It turns out that a number of different cytokines,

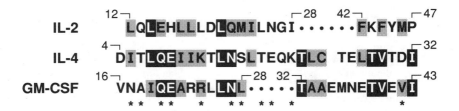

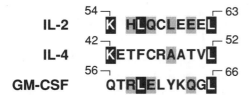

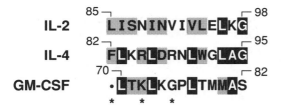

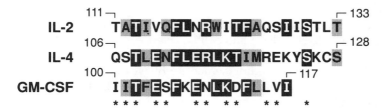

FIGURE 3-11 Sequence comparison of IL-2, IL-4, and GM-CSF. Helix A is given first and helix D is given last.

certainly IL-2, IL-4, and IL-7 and possibly some others, share the gamma C (common gamma receptor) subunit (formerly called IL-2 gamma receptor). Some of these cytokines are involved in pathways that regulate the activity of other cytokines. For example, the IL-2 and IL-4 pathways are intertwined, and they also use some of the identical components. Influencing the levels of the common gamma subunit in hope of modifying the activity of IL-4 may also modify the activities of IL-2 and IL-7 in such a way that the result may be the opposite of what was intended.

It is obvious that this is a very difficult field. How do we go about even postulating how to make drugs that could modify the activity of these types of molecules? First, by just looking at mutants of the naturally occurring proteins and identifying which parts of the proteins are important. A particular mutation of IL-4, for example, converts tyrosine 124 into aspartic acid, producing a molecule that is a full antagonist of IL-4 (Kruse et al., 1992).

To explain the action of antagonists, we have to understand how these signaling molecules work. The accepted mechanism is that the signaling event must involve dimerization of the extracellular domains of the receptors, leading to dimerization of the respective intracellular domains and then to a very complicated cascade of events. The dimerization of the extracellular domain is crucial and can sometimes occur without cytokines (e.g., antibodies can sometimes dimerize the receptors). Molecules that bind to the receptors are antagonists. Binding to the first molecule of the receptors but preventing the binding of the second molecule would prevent dimerization. In the case of tyrosine-124 mutant of IL-4, the specific receptor activity is not affected at all by this mutation but the biological activity is affected. We expect that this particular residue must interact with the common gamma subunit. A similar situation was reported for IL-2: a mutation of glutamine 126 into aspartic acid (Imler and Zurawski, 1992). Clearly this part of the structure is crucial to proper signaling by both cytokines.

Experimental structures of these complexes are not available, and we had to resort to modeling (Figure 3-13, see color plate). Unfortunately, it turns out that tyrosine 124 seems to be pointing halfway between the two receptor molecules, so trying to decide on which side to put the gamma receptor and on which side to put the IL-4 receptor is not obvious. However, some indirect interactions may be taking place. The residue arginine 121 corresponds to the glutamine in IL-2, which seems to be have properties similar to those of the mutant IL-4. So, mutation may be influencing the binding indirectly rather than directly.

Regardless of the interaction, modification of this area of the molecule may produce potential leads for drugs. However, drugs that are proteins are not very good because they cannot be given orally and are suitable only for conditions that are severe enough to warrant drugs given by injection. Of course, the next step would be to try to design small molecules that would correspond to the epitopes that are involved in receptor binding, thus antagonizing cytokines. We are still quite a long way from being able to go from these structures of proteins to the structure of small molecules that would replace those proteins.

In the long run, the approach described for cytokines may turn out to be important for the pharmacology of the future. We do not know today how to accomplish the goals, but sometimes posing questions is very important, even if there are no easy answers.

REFERENCES

Bazan, J. F. 1990. Structural design and molecular evolution of a cytokine receptor super-family. Proc. Natl. Acad. Sci. USA 87:6934-6938.

de Vos, A. M., M. Ultsch, and A. A. Kossiakoff. 1992. Human growth hormone and extracellular domain of its receptor: crystal structure of the complex. Science 255:306-312.

Imler, J.-L., and G. Zurawski. 1992. Receptor binding and internalization of mouse interleukin-2 derivatives that are partial agonists. J. Biol. Chem. 267:13185-13190.

Kruse, N., H.-P. Tony, and W. Swbold. 1992. Conversion of human interleukin-4 into a high affinity antagonist by a single amino acid repacement. EMBO J. 11:3237-3244.

Lam, P. Y. S., P. K. Jadhav, C. J. Eyermann, C. N. Hodge, Y. Ru, L. T. Bacheler, J. L., Meek, M. J. Otto, M. M. Rayner, Y. N. Wong, C.-H. Chang, P. C. Weber, D. A. Jackson, T. R. Sharpe, and S. Erickson-Viitanen. 1994. Rational design of potent, bioavailable, non-petide cyclic ureas as HIV protease inhibitors. Science 263:380-384.

Russell, S. M., A. D. Keegan, N. Harada, Y. Nakamura, M. Noguchi, P. Leland, M. C. Friedmann, A. Miyajima, R. K. Pure, W. E. Paul, and W. J. Leonard. 1993. Interleukin-2 receptor γ chain: a functional component of the interleukin-4 receptor. Science 262: 1880-1883.

4

The Future of Biotechnology

C. THOMAS CASKEY

The technology that has evolved since the discovery of the structure of the DNA molecule will drive many of the opportunities that exist in medicine, society, and industry. We must be careful in evaluating the technology and the information that comes from it so that we make wise societal decisions.

HIGHLIGHTS OF RECENT DISCOVERIES

From the time line of the discoveries in this field in the past 30 or more years (Figure 4-1, Table 4-1), we can see that advances were made rapidly. Discovery and use of bacterial restriction enzymes (Kelly and Smith, 1970; Smith and Wilcox, 1970) and the development of plasmid technology (Cohen et al., 1973) meant that complex molecules of DNA could be dissected into small elements and analyzed individually.

Ed Southern (1975) gave us the first technique for diagnosis via a molecular method. This technique was DNA-based and could detect specific regions of DNA even when diluted 10^8-fold. We had not previously seen such sensitive technology in medicine. Two other marvelous techniques in the 1970s were the independent discoveries of methods for sequencing DNA (Maxam and Gilbert, 1977; Sanger et al., 1977). These methods enabled us to look at base sequences in DNA. Then in the 1980s, the polymerase chain reaction (PCR) technology came out of the biotech industry, from the Cetus Corporation (Mullis et al., 1986; Saiki et al., 1985). PCR enabled us to dissect the human genome efficiently by work-

43

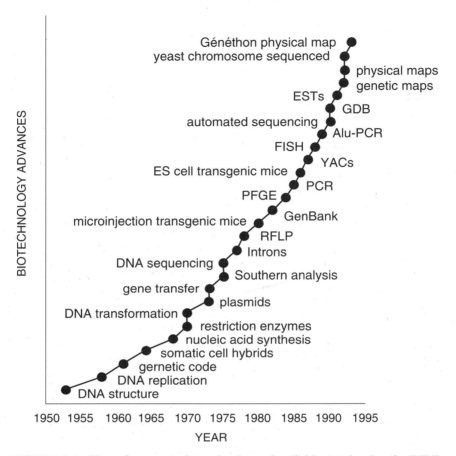

BIOTECHNOLOGY ADVANCES

- Généthon physical map
- yeast chromosome sequenced
- physical maps
- genetic maps
- ESTs
- GDB
- automated sequencing
- Alu-PCR
- FISH
- YACs
- ES cell transgenic mice
- PCR
- PFGE
- GenBank
- microinjection transgenic mice
- RFLP
- Introns
- DNA sequencing
- Southern analysis
- gene transfer
- plasmids
- DNA transformation
- restriction enzymes
- nucleic acid synthesis
- somatic cell hybrids
- gernetic code
- DNA replication
- DNA structure

1950 1955 1960 1965 1970 1975 1980 1985 1990 1995

YEAR

FIGURE 4-1 Key advances in biotechnology. See Table 4-1 for details. RFLP, restriction fragment length polymorphism; PFGE, purified field gel electrophoresis; PCR, polymerase chain reaction; ES, embryonic stem; YAC, yeast artificial chromosomes; FISH, fluorescence in situ hybridization; GDB, Genome Data Base; EST, expressed sequence tag.

ing with large cloned molecules. We could now clone elements of DNA up to 1 million base pairs long, which was much longer than the few thousand base pairs contained within a plasmid (Burke et al., 1987). Another highlight was the remarkable integration of technology using PCR and common sequences within the human genome to enable us to lift sequences easily and rapidly out of a very complex molecule, such as the yeast artificial chromosome (Olson et al., 1989).

The introduction of genome and sequence databases occurred in the

TABLE 4-1 Biotechnology Advances

Advances	Year	Referemce
X-ray structure of DNA determined	1953	Watson and Crick
Mechanism of DNA replication in *E. coli* determined	1958	Meselson and Stahl
Genetic code elucidated	1961	Nirenberg and Matthaei
Somatic cell hybrids generated	1964	Littlefield
Mechanism of nucleic acid synthesis determined	1968	Okazaki et al.
First restriction endonuclease isolated	1970	Smith and Wilcox, Kelly and Smith
DNA transformed into *E. coli*	1970	Mandel and Higa
Molecular cloning in plasmids achieved	1973	Cohen et al.
Gene transferred into cells	1973	McBride and Ozer
Southern analysis	1975	Southern
DNA sequenced	1975	Sanger and Coulson
Introns within genes discovered	1977	Breathnach et al.
Restriction fragment length polymorphisms (RFLPs) used	1978	Kan and Dozy
Transgenic mice generated from microinjected embryos	1980	Gordon et al.
GenBank established	1982	
Pulsed-field gel electrophoresis performed	1984	Schwartz and Cantor
Polymerase chain reaction performed	1985	Saiki et al., Mullis et al.
Transgenic mice generated from embryonal stem cells	1986	Robertson et al.
Yeast artificial chromosomes cloned	1987	Burke et al.
Fluorescence in situ hybridization performed	1988	Lawrence et al.
Alu polymerase chain reaction performed	1989	Nelson et al.
Automated sequencing of *HPRT* gene performed	1990	Edwards et al.
Genome Data Base (GDB) established	1990	
Expressed sequence tags created	1991	Adams et al.
Genetic map of all human chromosomes created	1992	NIH/CEPH Collaborative Mapping Group
Physical maps of human chromosomes 21 and Y created	1992	Chumakov et al., Foote et al., Vollrath et al.
Yeast chromosome III sequenced	1992	Oliver et al.
Généthon physical map developed	1993	Cohen et al.

1980s. An investigator anywhere could sit down at a computer and have access to data being generated worldwide. Then came the development of genetic and physical maps of the human genome. In 1993 came the announcement by the Généthon group in Paris of the development of a genetic linkage map containing more than 2,000 markers (Cohen et al., 1993). This map essentially fulfilled one of the short-term mapping goals of the Human Genome Project 1 year before the target date (U.S. Department of Health and Human Services and Department of Energy, 1990).

THE HUMAN GENOME PROJECT

Scientists working on the Human Genome Project have developed a set of markers along each chromosome that enable them to quickly and easily map regions of the genome and then actually isolate the material. The linear order of the material is then determined so that the chromosome can be reconstructed.

A new development in the Human Genome Project is the ability to seek disease genes. There are an estimated 80,000 genes in the human genome, of which about 2,000 have been isolated (McKusick et al., 1994). The ultimate goal of the Human Genome Project, determining the base sequence of the human genome, is currently beyond our available technology. However, identifying and characterizing all human genes (approximately 3 percent of the total sequence) is fully within our capacity.

We are adding entries to McKusick et al.'s (1994) *Mendelian Inheritance of Man* at an increasing pace, but this is still slow compared with what will be seen in the next few years. About 5 percent of the estimated 80,000 genes have been mapped, and at least 770 cloned and mapped genes have been associated with clinical abnormalities. Disease genes are found by looking for abnormal genes in affected patients. This process, however, will change with the increased discovery of genes. In the future, newly isolated genes will be studied and then patients will be found who fit their characteristics.

TRINUCLEOTIDE REPEAT DISEASES

The discovery of a gene can lead to insights into a previously unknown system. The fragile X syndrome is so called because under certain culture conditions affected X chromosomes break at the q27.3 region, near the end of the long arm. Fragile X syndrome is the most common form of inherited mental retardation worldwide. From observing chromosomal breakage in culture and then tracking genome markers through affected families, we knew that the gene or genes responsible for this disease resided in Xq27.3. Classical positional cloning technology, used to iden-

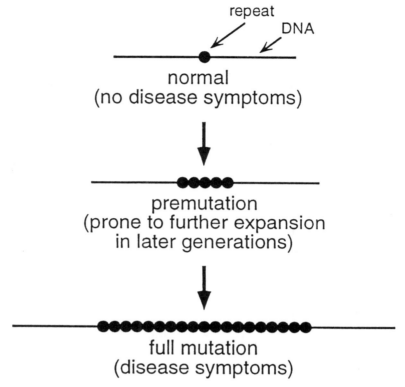

repeat
DNA

normal
(no disease symptoms)

premutation
(prone to further expansion
in later generations)

full mutation
(disease symptoms)

FIGURE 4-2 Expansion of unstable repeat regions resulting in disease. Some disease genes contain a region of repeated triplet nucleotides that is polymorphic (that is, the number of repeats is variable). Reproduced with permission from Rossiter and Caskey (In Press).

tify the gene, revealed that a new form of mutation was found at the site of a variable trinucleotide repeat (Verkerk et al., 1991) (Figure 4-2). All of us have a few cytosine-cytosine-guanine trinucleotide repeats at this location, but children with the mental retardation syndrome have markedly expanded trinucleotide repeats (Fu et al., 1991). The expanded trinucleotide repeats are very unstable when transmitted from generation to generation. Never before had we seen such unstable DNA that rendered such a high susceptibility to disease.

A recent study analyzed individual molecules of DNA from the sperm of an asymptomatic male for a disease called myotonic dystrophy (Monckton et al., 1995). This disease is also caused by unstable trinucleotide repeats. The size of the repeat region in the man's blood cells was 75

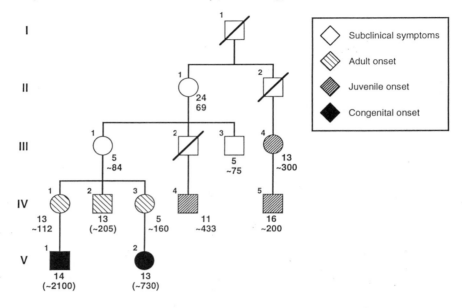

FIGURE 4-3 Myotonic dystrophy pedigree, showing trinucleotide repeat expansion. The number of $(GCT)_n$ repeats in each allele is given for each individual in this five-generation pedigree. The upper number is the normal allele and the lower number is the expanded allele. This family illustrates the phenomenon of trinucleotide expansion but also has one of the rare examples of a reduction in size of the repeat region (from III-4 to IV-5). Reproduced with permission from Monckton and Caskey (1995).

units, which caused him no health difficulty. However, the size of the repeat region in his sperm ranged from 30 to 450 units. Larger repeat sizes tend to result in more severe disease (Redman et al., 1993).

The fragile X syndrome and myotonic dystrophy findings were new discoveries in human genetics. They constitute molecular understanding of what clinicians for years had called "anticipation," the increase in severity and earlier onset of disease in later generations (Fu et al., 1991). Figure 4-3 shows an example of expansion of a trinucleotide repeat within a myotonic dystrophy family. As the repeat region expands from generation to generation, the disease appears in a more severe form. This family was unaware of their myotonic dystrophy until the birth of individual V-1. His cousin had died as a newborn after 10 days on a respirator, but her myotonic dystrophy was not recognized.

How many other trinucleotide repeat diseases are there? At the moment we know of spinal and bulbar muscular atrophy, two forms of fragile X mental retardation, myotonic dystrophy, Huntington disease,

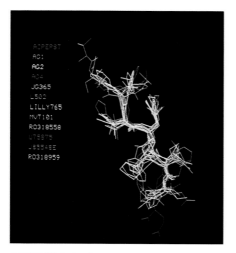

FIGURE 3-6   Superposition of the structures of several inhibitors of HIV proteas.

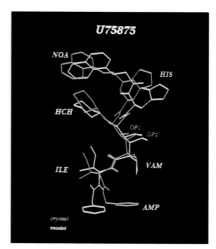

FIGURE 3-7   Modeled and experimental structures of U75875.

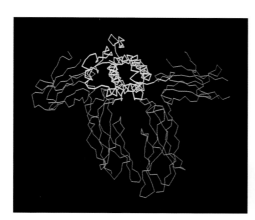

FIGURE 3-9   Interaction of human growth hormone with its receptor.

FIGURE 3-10   Superpositions of IL-2, IL-4, and GM-CSF.

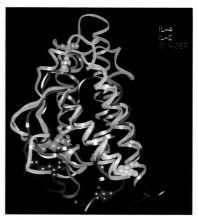

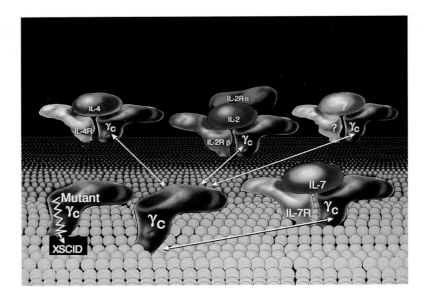

FIGURE 3-12   Common receptors of cytokines.

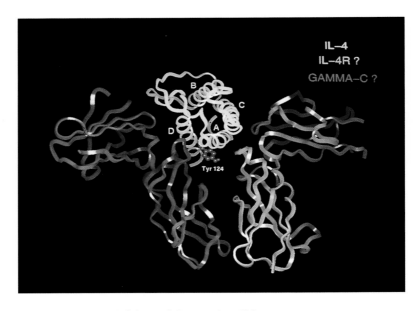

FIGURE 3-13   Modeling of eht tyrosine-124 mutant.

spinocerebellar ataxia type 1, dentatorubral-pallidoluysian atrophy, and Machado-Joseph disease (Willems, 1994). All these diseases are neurological disorders, but whether this is significant is not known.

DIAGNOSTIC PROCEDURES

Physicians and patients can benefit from the accuracy and precision in diagnosis provided by genetic diagnostic procedures. In the future this information may enable us to intervene by medication or lifestyle alterations to preempt the onset of a disease in a person at risk. Accurate diagnosis will identity couples at risk for bearing children affected by a genetic disease.

Duchenne muscular dystrophy is a common and severe childhood disease. The dystrophin gene, responsible for the disease, is very large and is particularly prone to deletion mutations (Clemens and Caskey, 1992), and most patients do not have the same deletion. Scanning the huge dystrophin gene may seem to be an impossibility but in fact is very simple. By using PCR technology, many regions of the gene can be analyzed simultaneously and more than 98 percent of deletions can be detected with a simple procedure called multiplex PCR (Chamberlain et al., 1990) (Figure 4-4). Multiplex PCR analysis has proved to be readily transferable to clinical laboratories worldwide, a particular benefit for laboratories that could not afford the more complex diagnostic procedures used previously (Group study, 1992).

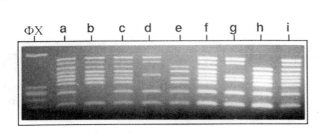

Order	
Exon	Size (bp)
45	547
48	506
19	459
17	416
51	388
8	360
12	331
44	268
4	196

FIGURE 4-4 Scanning for deletions in the Duchenne muscular dystrophy gene. Nine fragments from the dystrophin gene (lanes a,c,f,i) are generated by simultaneous polymerase chain reactions and separated by size. The absence of one or more bands (lanes b,d,e,g,h) indicates that there is a deletion of that portion of the dystrophin gene. This method is used for diagnosing Duchenne muscular dystrophy at Baylor College of Medicine and many other institutions. Reproduced with permission from [study group] (1992).

A second example of improved diagnosis followed the discovery of the cystic fibrosis gene, responsible for the most common recessively inherited disease in Caucasians (Beaudet, 1992). The diagnostic problem with cystic fibrosis is that many (more than 300) disease-causing mutations have been identified throughout the gene. Just as Duchenne muscular dystrophy required a scanning method of deletion detection, cystic fibrosis requires a method of scanning for small (mostly single base pair) alterations. We are doing this by using a robot to analyze 22 different positions in the gene. In a single assay, one technician can run up to 90 samples. Thus, molecular diagnosis for cystic fibrosis has rapidly moved from research to general use at a reasonable cost. Families can find out if they have a risk for this disease before bearing a child with cystic fibrosis. Or, if they have a child with cystic fibrosis, they can find out who else in the family is at risk and what their future reproductive options are.

The Human Genome Project is a very ambitious project that has the capacity to identify significant disease risks in all of us. Every individual probably carries 5 to 10 significant genetic mutations with the potential to cause severe disease at various stages of life. In several laboratories a "chip" technology is being developed that will scan large portions of the genome for mutations (Fodor et al., 1993). Attached to a chip would be DNA sequences that correspond to the sites of mutations for common diseases. A person's DNA could then be hybridized to that chip and the resulting signal would indicate which mutations were found. It is possible to place 100 or more DNA molecules on a single 1-centimeter chip and to use a detection device to read those signals. It is going to be possible with this or a similar technology to look at targeted regions of the genome and diagnose a disease or determine susceptibility for bearing an affected child.

POSSIBILITIES FOR DISEASE PREVENTION

How these diagnostic advances can be used to prevent disease will affect how we view health care and what we will allow to take place in our society. For example, let us consider alpha-1-antitrypsin deficiency, type II hyperlipidemia, Huntington disease, and certain types of cancer. These are all diseases in which it is possible to run a DNA-based analysis and determine if a person has the DNA alteration that is going to lead to the disease. Each of these diseases has a different time of onset in life, but the diagnostic test can be done at any age.

Alpha-1-antitrypsin deficiency is a common cause of adult-onset emphysema (Blank and Brantly, 1994). If you knew from birth that you had this deficiency and if you abstained from smoking, you would prolong your life by 10 years (Larsson, 1978). This is an example of a lifestyle choice improving the outcome of a condition that is determined genetically.

Coronary artery disease is a major killer in the United States and one that has received a lot of attention, but most of the focus has been on treatment after the disease develops. However, detection of a genetic predisposition to hypercholesterolemia permits intervention with diet and medication before the damage is bad enough to cause symptoms (Bild et al., 1993).

Not all presymptomatic diagnosis has the option of treatment. Huntington disease, a devastating neurological disorder, can be diagnosed very precisely by using DNA methods (Huntington's Disease Collaborative Research Group, 1993). However, at present there is no treatment or cure. Because of the dominant inheritance of this gene, any child with an affected parent has a 50 percent chance of possessing the same defective gene. For Huntington disease, presymptomatic testing might help in eliminating uncertainty and planning the future, but there is no option for improving health. This will also be true for other diseases until we have a greater understanding of mechanisms of disease and have developed better therapeutic measures.

Numerous genes throughout the genome are responsible for predisposing an individual to developing cancer (Figure 4-5). Recently discovered genes include those that contribute to breast and colon cancer. Offspring of parents with cancer live in uncertainty, not knowing whether or not that predisposition has been inherited. In the future there will be less uncertainty. However, this information must be handled carefully. Are you prepared to learn whether you are at high risk for developing cancer? What effect would that have on your life? What would your doctors do? These are issues to which we will be increasingly exposed as presymptomatic diagnosis becomes more accurate and commonly used.

PRIVACY ISSUES

What is the potential down side to this prior information? There may be loss of privacy resulting from increased knowledge about your future medical condition. You and your physician will now share some information that was previously unknown. How many others would you want to share that information with? Your spouse? Your children? Your siblings? These would all seem rather logical to me. Perhaps you have an employment health care plan that requires you to report any health difficulties. Is it possible that information might begin to slip from that ultimate privacy between you and physician? I would say yes.

Although many people would argue strongly that we have to protect the privacy of an individual's genetic information, I would argue a slightly

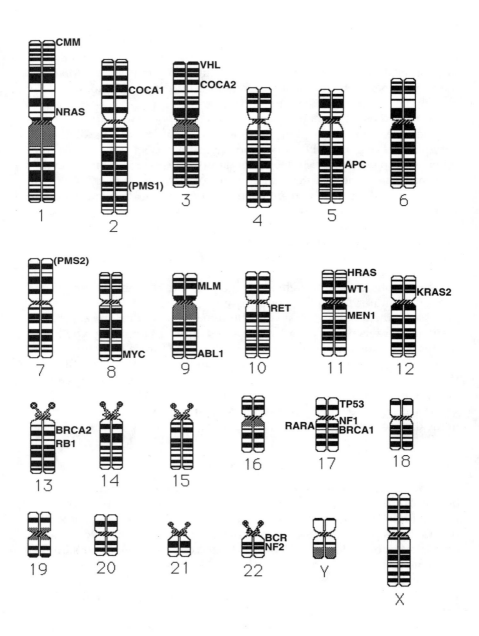

different point. I am going to accept that this information might become widespread and argue that we should make sure that there is no ill effect from this acquired information (e.g., exclusion from insurance, employment, education, or other opportunities). An individual's rights should be protected. I think this would be a more logical way to proceed in what I think is going to be an increasingly open society regarding information. Many disagree with this and insist that such information be kept private, but I have worked in medicine and dealt with families for too long to think that privacy can be achieved. Therefore, the protection of the information against misuse is very important.

Everyone carries some genetic error; some have a few illnesses and others are spared sickness. The only way that we can support the total societal burden of illness is to have a uniform underwriting of the entire population. The healthy people have to pay for the ill health of the rare individuals in the population. It is extremely important that we be able to gain access to presymptomatic information without damage to the patient, so that we can implement new procedures for disease prevention in the future.

DRUG PRODUCTION

Genetic research has also affected the area of drug production. In the past, insulin could only be obtained from abattoir material, growth hormone was extracted from cadaver brains, and clotting factor VIII was prepared from pooled blood. Cellular growth factors were not available until the era of recombinant DNA. All of these now can be produced very effectively by industry by using recombinant DNA techniques.

FIGURE 4-5 (opposite) Genomic location of some genes involved in human cancer. ABL1, Abelson murine leukemia viral (v-*abl*) oncogene homolog 1; APC, adenomatosis polyposis coli; BCR, breakpoint cluster region (chronic myeloid leukemia); BRCA1, breast cancer 1, early onset; CMM, cutaneous malignant melanoma/dysplastic nevus; COCA1, colon cancer 1; HRAS, Harvey rat sarcoma viral (v-Ha-*ras*) oncogene homolog; KRAS2, Kirsten rat sarcoma 2 viral (v-Ki-*ras*2) oncogene homolog; MEN1, multiple endocrine neoplasia 1; MLM, melanoma; MYC, Avian myelocytomatosis viral (v-*myc*) oncogene homolog; NF1, neurofibromin 1 (neurofibromatosis, von Recklinghausen disease, Watson disease); NF2, neurofibromastosis 2 (bilateral acoustic neuroma); NRAS, neuroblastoma RAS viral (v-*ras*) oncogene homolog; RARA, retinoic acid receptor, alpha; RB1, retinoblastoma 1 (including osteosarcoma); RET, ret proto-oncogene (multiple endocrine neoplasia MEN2A and medullary thyroid carcinoma 1, and Hirschsprung disease); TP53, tumor protein p53 (Li-Fraumeni syndrome); VHL, von Hippel-Lindau syndrome; and WT1, Wilms tumor 1. Redrawn from Caskey and Smith (1994).

Despite early resistance to the use of genetic engineering techniques, these methods have proved lifesaving in many situations. Virtually all hemophilia A patients who were treated before 1985 with factor VIII made from blood now carry the human immunodeficiency virus or have died from acquired immune disease syndrome. Another common complication is hepatitis resulting from contaminating viruses. However, the ability to make factor VIII from an isolated gene has eliminated the use of blood products and the problem of viral contamination (Kaufman, 1989). Another example of a disease caused by contamination of therapeutic materials with infectious agents is Creutzfeldt-Jakob disease, a neurodegenerative disease leading to dementia and death. Some people taking growth hormone made from the brains of cadavers have contracted this disease. Again, the growth factor is now manufactured from an isolated gene (Goeddel et al., 1979).

Many recombinant drugs are coming onto the market. It is important that these drugs undergo careful clinical evaluation to determine their utility and efficacy. They are powerful drugs with tremendous utility in certain settings, but it is very important to prove their clinical application before they move into the marketplace. We cannot automatically accept drugs just because they are recombinant drugs; they must earn their place in the medical armament.

GENE THERAPY

Gene therapy is a technology that will have a major effect on the practice of medicine. In most cases the chosen delivery system is a viral vector that has been disabled. The essential functions are removed from the virus and replaced with DNA sequences that correspond to the human disease of interest. The engineered virus can then be safely produced in large quantities and used for delivering those genes (McCabe, 1993).

One disease that is a candidate for gene therapy is the severe combined immune deficiency resulting from deficiency in the enzyme adenosine deaminase. Bone marrow transplantation can be used to treat this disease but is limited by the availability of matched donors and the problems associated with immune-rejection reactions. At least two young girls have been successfully provided with functional adenosine deaminase genes, enabling them to lead relatively normal lives instead of being kept in complete isolation (Blaese et al., 1994).

In our laboratory we are developing gene therapy for a common liver disease called ornithine transcarbamylase deficiency. Mice with an equivalent of this disease have no hair and are therefore easily distinguished. These mice can be completely corrected by a single injection given in the newborn period of a virus carrying the ornithine transcarbamylase gene (M. A. Morsy, T. Ngo, A. W. Warman, W. E. O'Brien, F. L. Graham, and C. T. Caskey, unpublished data). This is an example of gene therapy administered once that results in a cure in mice. This form of treatment is permanent and blood borne and is probably going to be the future direction for gene therapy, although the vector may not necessarily be a virus.

GENETIC PERSONAL IDENTIFICATION

Personal identification based on genetic information is currently used in cases involving paternity, missing individuals, and forensic evidence. It is also used extensively by population geneticists. It is estimated that any two people will have differences in DNA structure in about 1 nucleotide per 300 to 1,000 (Cooper et al., 1985). Huge diversity exists in the population, and it is this variation in DNA structure that is used for personal identification.

Let me use forensic analysis in a rape case to illustrate the method (Gill et al., 1985). A DNA sample from the victim is obtained from blood and also from the secretions taken when the victim seeks medical attention. Male and female fractions from the vaginal sample can be separated, resulting in distinctive DNA signals. Eyewitness accounting of violent crimes is notoriously inaccurate, but this DNA "fingerprinting" precisely demonstrates a match or mismatch between a suspect and biological material left at the scene of a crime. Several regions of the genome are scanned during the analysis by using different genetic probes. With each probe that displays a match between two samples, the statistical probability that they came from the same person is increased. If a mismatch is shown, the samples cannot have come from the same individual. This is a very powerful technique, particularly when used to prove innocence.

The use of DNA fingerprinting was fought extensively in the courts at the federal and local levels, but technology has now withstood the test of time through the court systems. It was reviewed carefully by the National Academy of Sciences, which issued guidelines on how this technology should be used in the courts (Committee on DNA Technology in Forensic Science, 1992). This technology has also been used in archeological digs to solve crimes of many years ago. The Romanov family assassinations that took place in Russia have now been clarified by this technology (Debenham, 1994; Gill et al., 1994).

DNA variation can also be used to investigate the migration of human populations in the past (Torroni et al., 1994). Such studies have taken advantage of the fact that there is sequence variation in mitochondrial DNA and that mitochondrial DNA is inherited entirely from the mother.

DNA analysis will enable us to discover (and hopefully understand) our genes and identify those that cause disease. The capture of some genes will enable us to develop pharmaceutical agents that can benefit individuals with disease. The use of this technology will enable us to better understand our past and our diversity.

REFERENCES

Adams, M. D., J. M. Kelley, J. D. Gocayne, M. Dubnick, M. H. Polymeropolous, H. Xiao, C. R. Merril, A. Wu, B. Olde, R. F. Moreno, A. R. Kerlavage, W. R. McCombie, and J. C. Venter. 1991. Complementary DNA sequencing: expressed sequence tags and Human Genome Project. Science 252:1651-1656.

Beaudet, A. L. 1992. Genetic testing for cystic fibrosis. Pediatr. Clin. North Am. 39:213-228.

Bild, D. E., R. R. Williams, H. B. Brewer, J. A. Herd, T. A. Pearson, and E. Stein. 1993. Identification and management of heterozygous familial hypercholesterolemia: summary and recommendations from an NHLBI workshop. Am. J. Cardiol. 72:1D-5D.

Blaese, R. M., K. Culver, W. F. Anderson, J. Ramsey, C. Carter, A. D. Miller, C. Mullen, D. Kohn, and R. Morgan. 1994. Gene therapy for adenosine deaminase (ADA) deficiency: a 4 year follow-up of the original trial. P.3 in Abstracts of papers presented at the 1994 meeting on gene therapy, September 21-September 25, 1994, T. Friedmann, Y. W. Kan, and R. Mulligan, eds. Cold Spring Harbor, NY: Cold Spring Harbor Laboratory.

Blank, C. A., and M. Brantly. 1994. Clinical features and molecular characteristics of alpha 1-antitrypsin deficiency. Ann. Allergy 72:105-120.

Breathnach, R., J. L. Mandel, and P. Chambon. 1977. Ovalbumin gene is split in chicken DNA. Nature 270:314-319.

Burke, D. T., G. F. Carle, and M. V. Olson. 1987. Cloning of large segments of exogenous DNA into yeast by means of artificial chromosome vectors. Science 236:806-812.

Caskey, C. T., and J. M. Smith. 1994. Sizing up the enemy. A call for papers on cancer [editorial]. JAMA 271:1448-1449.

Chamberlain, J. S., R. A. Gibbs, J. E. Rainer, and C. T. Caskey. 1990. Multiplex PCR for the diagnosis of Duchenne muscular dystrophy. Pp. 272-281 in PCR Protocols: A Guide to Methods and Applications, M. Innis, D. Gelfand, J. Sninsky, and T. White, eds. Orlando, FL: Academic Press.

Chumakov, I., P. Rigault, S. Guillou, P. Ougen, A. Billaut, G. Guasconi, P. Gervy, I. LeGall, P. Soularue, L. Grinas, L. Bougueleret, C. Bellanné-Chantelot, B. Lacroix, E. Barillot, P. Gesnouin, S. Pook, G. Vaysseix, G. Frelat, A. Schmitz, J. L. Sambucy, A. Bosch, X. Estivill, J. Weissenbach, A. Vignal, H. Riethman, D. Cox, D. Patterson, K. Gardiner, M. Hattori, Y. Sakai, H. Ichikawa, M. Ohki, D. le Paslier, R. Heilig, S. Antonarakis, and D. Cohen. 1992. Continuum of overlapping clones spanning the entire human chromosome 21q. Nature 359:380-387.

Clemens, P. R., and C. T. Caskey. 1992. Duchenne muscular dystrophy. Curr Neurol. 12:1-22.

Cohen, D., I. Chumakov, and J. Weissenbach. 1993. A first-generation physical map of the human genome. Nature 366:698-701.

Cohen, S. N., A. C. Y. Chang, H. W. Boyer, and R. B. Helling. 1973. Construction of biologically functional bacterial plasmids in vitro. Proc. Natl. Acad. Sci. USA 70:3240-3244.

Committee on DNA Technology in Forensic Science, Board on Biology, Commission on Life Science, and National Research Council. 1992. DNA Technology in Forensic Science. Washington, D.C.: National Academy Press.

Cooper, D. N., B. A. Smith, H. J. Cook, S. Niemann, and J. Schmidtke. 1985. An estimate of unique DNA sequence heterozygosity in the human genome. Hum. Genet. 69:201-205.

Debenham, P. G. 1994. Genetics leaves no bones unturned. Nat. Genet. 6:113-114.

Edwards, A., H. Voss, P. Rice, A. Civitello, J. Stegemann, C. Schwager, J. Zimmermann, H. Erfle, C. T. Caskey, and W. Ansorge. 1990. Automated DNA sequencing of the human HPRT locus. Genomics 6:593-608.

Fodor, S. P. A., R. P. Rava, X. C. Huang, A. C. Pease, C. P. Holmes, and C. L. Adams. 1993. Multiplexed biochemical assays with biological chips. Nature 364:555-556.

Foote, S., D. Vollrath, A. Hilton, and D. C. Page. 1992. The human Y chromosome: overlapping DNA clones spanning the euchromatic region. Science 258:60-66.

Fu, Y. H., D. P. A. Kuhl, A. Pizzuti, M. Pieretti, J. S. Sutcliffe, S. Richards, A. J. M. H. Verkerkk, J. J. A. Holden, R. G. Fenwick, Jr., S. T. Warren, B. A. Oostra, D. L. Nelson, and C. T. Caskey. 1991. Variation of the CGG repeat at the fragile X site results in genetic instability: resolution of the Sherman paradox. Cell 67:1047-1048.

Gill P., A. J. Jeffreys, and D. J. Werrett. 1985. Forensic application of DNA 'fingerprints.' Nature 318:577-579.

Gill, P., P. L. Ivanov, C. Kimpton, R. Piercy, N. Benson, G. Tully, I. Evett, E. Hagelberg, and K. Sullivan. 1994. Identification of the remains of the Romanov family by DNA analysis. Nat. Genet. 6:130-135.

Goeddel, D. V., H. L. Heyneker, T. Hozumi, R. Arentzen, K. Itakura, D. G. Yansura, M. J. Ross, G. Miozzari, R. Crea, and P. H. Seeburg. 1979. Direct expression in *Escherichia coli* of a DNA sequence coding for human growth hormone. Nature 281:544-548.

Gordon, J. W., G. A. Scangos, D. J. Plotkin, J. A. Barbosa, and F. H. Ruddle. 1980. Genetic transformation of mouse embryos by microinjection of purified DNA. Proc. Natl. Acad. Sci. USA 77:7380-7384.

Group study. 1992. Diagnosis of Duchenne and Becker muscular dystrophies by polymerase chain reaction. A multicenter study. JAMA 267:2609-2615.

Huntington's Disease Collaborative Research Group. 1993. A novel gene containing a trinucleotide repeat that is expanded and unstable on Huntington's disease chromosomes. Cell 72:971-983.

Kan, Y. W., and A. M. Dozy. 1978. Polymorphism of DNA sequence adjacent to human b-globin structural gene: relationship to sickle mutation. Proc. Natl. Acad. Sci. USA 75:5631-5635.

Kaufman, R. J. 1989. Genetic engineering of factor VIII. Nature 342:207-208.

Kelly, T. J., Jr., and H. O. Smith. 1970. A restriction enzyme from *Hemophilus influenzae*. II. Base sequence of the recognition site. J. Mol. Biol. 51:393-409.

Larsson, C. 1978. Natural history and life expectancy in severe alpha$_1$-antitrypsin deficiency, Pi Z. Acta Med. Scand. 204:345-351.

Lawrence, J. B., C. A. Villnave, and R. H. Singer. 1988. Sensitive, high resolution chromatin and chromosome mapping in situ: presence and orientation of two closely integrated copies of EBV in a lymphoma line. Cell 52:51-61.

Littlefield, J. W. 1964. Selection of hybrids from matings of fibroblasts in vitro and their presumed recombinants. Science 145:709-710.

Mandel, M., and A. Higa. 1970. Calcium-dependent bacteriophage DNA infection. J. Mol. Biol. 53:159-162.

Maxam, A. M., and W. Gilbert. 1977. A new method for sequencing DNA. Proc. Natl. Acad. Sci. USA 74:560-564.

McBride, O. W., and H. L. Ozer. 1973. Transfer of genetic information by purified metaphase chromosomes. Proc. Natl. Acad. Sci. USA 70:1258-1262.

McCabe, E. R. B. 1993. Clinical application of gene therapy: emerging opportunities and current limitations. Biochem. Med. Metab. Biol. 50:241-253.

McKusick, V. A., C. A. Francomano, S. E. Antonarakis, and P. L. Pearson. 1994. Mendelian Inheritance in Man. A Catalog of Human Genes and Genetic Disorders, 11th edition. Baltimore, MD: Johns Hopkins University Press.

Meselson, M., and F. W. Stahl. 1958. The replication of DNA in *Escherichia coli*. Proc. Natl. Acad. Sci. USA 44:671-682.

Monckton, D. G., and C. T. Caskey. 1995. Unstable triplet repeat diseases. Circulation 91:513-520.

Monckton, D. G., L. J. C. Wong, T. Ashizawa, and C. T. Caskey. 1995. Somatic mosaicism, germline expansions, germline reversions and intergenerational reductions in myotonic dystrophy males: small pool PCR analyses. Hum. Mol. Genet. 4:1-8.

Mullis, K., F. Faloona, S. Scharf, R. Saiki., G. Horn, and H. Erlich. 1986. Specific enzymatic amplification of DNA in vitro: the polymerase chain reaction. Cold Spring Harb. Symp. Quant. Biol. 51:263-273.

Nelson, D. L., S. A. Ledbetter, L. Corbo, M. F. Victoria, R. Ramirez-Solis, T. D. Webster, D. H. Ledbetter, and C. T. Caskey. 1989. *Alu* polymerase chain reaction: a method for rapid isolation of human-specific sequences from complex DNA sources. Proc. Natl. Acad. Sci. USA 86:6686-6690.

NIH/CEPH Collaborative Mapping Group. 1992. A comprehensive genetic linkage map of the human genome. Science 258:67-86.

Nirenberg, M. W., and J. H. Matthaei. 1961. The dependence of cell-free protein synthesis in *E. coli* upon naturally occurring or synthetic polyribonucleotides. Proc. Natl. Acad. Sci. USA 47:1588-1602.

Okazaki, R., T. Okazaki, K. Sakabe, K. Sugimoto, and A. Sugino. 1968. Mechanism of DNA chain growth. I. Possible discontinuity and unusual secondary structure of newly synthesized chains. Proc. Natl. Acad. Sci. USA 59:598-605.

Oliver, S. G., Q. J. M. van der Aart, M. L. Agostoni-Carbone, M. Aigle, L. Alberghina, D. Alexandraki, G. Antoine, R. Anwar, J. P. G. Ballesta, P. Benit, G. Berben, E. Bergantino, N. Biteau, P. A. Bolle, M. Bolotin-Fukuhara, A. Brown, A. J. P. Brown, J. M. Buhler, C. Carcano, G. Carignani, H. Cederberg, R. Chanet, R. Contreras, M. Crouzet, B. Daignan-Fornier, E. Defoor, M. Delgado, J. Demolder, C. Doira, E. Dubois, B. Dujon, A. Dusterhoft, D. Erdmann, M. Esteban, F. Fabre, C. Fairhead, G. Faye, H. Feldmann, W. Fiers, M. C. Francingues-Gaillard, L. Franco, L. Frontali, H. Fukuhara, L. J. Fuller, P. Galland, M. E. Gent, D. Gigot, V. Gilliquet, N. Glansdorff, A. Goffeau, M. Grenson, P. Grisanti, L. A. Grivell, M. de Haan, M. Haasemann, D. Hatat, J. Hoenicka, J. Hegemann, C. . Herbert, F. Hilger, S. Hohmann, C. P. Hollenberg, K. Huse, F. Iborra, K. J. Indge, K. Isono, C. Jacq, M. Jacquet, C. M. James, J. C. Jauniaux, Y. Jia, A. Jimenez, A. Kelly, U. Kleinhans, P. Kreisi, G. Lanfranchi, C. Lewis, C. G. van der Linden, G. Lucchini, K. Lutzenkirchen, M. J. Maat, L. Mallet, G. Mannhaupt, E. Martegani, A. Mathieu, C. T. C. Maurer, D. McConnell, R. A. McKee, F. Messenguy, H. W. Mewes, F. Molemans, M. A. Montague, M. Muzi Falconi, L. Navas, C. S. Newlon, D. Noone, C. Pallier, L. Panzeri, B. M. Pearson, J. Perea, P. Philippsen, A. Pierard, R. J. Planta, P. Plevani, B. Poetsch, F. Pohl, B. Purnelle, M. Ramezani Rad, S. W. Rasmussen, A. Raynal, M. Remacha, P. Richterich, A. B. Roberts, F. Rodriguez, E. Sanz, I. Schaaff-Gerstenschlager, B. Scherens, B. Schweitzer, Y. Shu, J. Skala, P. P. Slonimski, F. Sor, C. Soustelle, R. Spiegelberg, L. I. Stateva, H. Y. Steensma, S. Steiner, A. Thierry, G. Thireos, M. Tzermia, L. A. Urrestauazu, B. Valle, I. R. Warmington, D. von Wettstein, B. L. Wixksteed, C. Wilson, H. Wurst, G. Xu, A. Yoshikawa, F. K. Zimmermann, and J. G. Sgouros. 1992. The complete DNA sequence of yeast chromosome III. Nature 357:38-46.

Olson, M., L. Hood, C. Cantor, and D. Botstein. 1989. A common language for physical mapping of the human genome. Science 245:1434-1435.

Redman, J. B., R. G. Fenwick, Jr., Y. H. Fu, A. Pizzuti, and C. T. Caskey. 1993. Relationship between parental trinucleotide GCT repeat length and severity of myotonic dystrophy in offspring. JAMA 269:1960-1965.

Robertson, E., A. Bradley, M. Kuehn, and M. Evans. 1986. Germ-line transmission of genes introduced into cultured pluripotential cells by retroviral vector. Nature 323:445-448.

Rossiter, B. J. F., and C. T. Caskey. In Press. Molecular biology of human genetic predisposition to disease In Encyclopedia of Molecular Biology and Biotechnology, R. A. Meyers, ed. Weinheim: VCH Publishers, in press.

Saiki, R. K., S. Scharf, F. Faloona, K. B. Mullis, G. T. Horn, H. A. Erlich, and N. Arnheim. 1985. Enzymatic amplification of b-globin genomic sequences and restriction site analysis for diagnosis of sickle cell anemia. Science. 230:1350-1354.

Sanger, F., and A. R. Coulson. 1975. A rapid method of determining sequences in DNA by primed synthesis with DNA polymerase. J. Mol. Biol. 94:441-448.

Sanger, F., S. Nicklen, and A. R. Coulson. 1977. DNA sequencing with chain-terminating inhibitors. Proc. Natl. Acad. Sci. USA 74:5463-5467.

Schwartz, D. C., and C. R. Cantor. 1984. Separation of yeast chromosome-sized DNAs by pulsed field gradient gel electrophoresis. Cell 37:67-75.

Smith, H. O., and K. W. Wilcox. 1970. A restriction enzyme from *Hemophilus influenzae*. I. Purification and general properties. J. Mol. Biol. 51:379-391.

Southern, E. M. 1975. Detection of specific sequences among DNA fragments separated by gel electrophoresis. J. Mol. Biol. 98:503-517.

Torroni, A., J. V. Neel, R. Barrantes, T. G. Schurr, and D. C. Wallace. 1994. Mitochondrial DNA "clock" for the Amerinds and its implications for timing their entry into North America. Proc. Natl. Acad. Sci. USA 91:1158-1162.

U.S. Department of Health and Human Services, and U.S. Department of Energy. 1990. Understanding Our Genetic Inheritance. The U.S. Human Genome Project: The First Five Years, FY 1991-1995. DOE/ER-0452P. Washington, D.C.: U.S. Government Printing Office.

Verkerk, A. J. M. H., M. Pieretti, J. S. Sutcliffe, Y. H. Fu, D. P. A. Kuhl, A. Pizutti, O. Reiner, S. Richards, M. F. Victoria, F. Zhang, B. E. Eussen, G. J. B. van Ommen, L. A. J. Blonden, G. J. Riggins, J. L. Chastain, C. . Kunst, H. Galjaard, C. T. Caskey, D. L. Nelson, B. A. Oostra, and S. T. Warren. 1991. Identification of a gene (*FMR-1*) containing a CGG repeat coincident with a breakpoint cluster region exhibiting length variation in fragile X syndrome. Cell 65:905-914.

Vollrath, D., S. Foote, A. Hilton, L. G. Brown, P. Beer-Romero, J. S. Bogan, and D. C. Page. 1992. The human Y chromosome: a 43-interval map based on naturally occurring deletions. Science 258:52-59.

Watson, J. D., and F. H. C. Crick. 1953. Molecular structure of nucleic acids. Nature 171:737-738.

Willems, P. J. 1994. Dynamic mutations hit double figures. Nat. Genet. 8:213-215.

Part 2

BIOTECHNOLOGY APPLICATIONS
TODAY AND TOMORROW

B iotechnology makes it possible to do things that previously lay in the realm of science fiction: manipulate genes, grow human tissues and organs outside the body, make endless supplies of drugs extracted from rare plants, destroy polluting chemicals. However, the road from experimental technology to reliable product is not always very smooth.

In this section, authors with expertise in different areas of biotechnology discuss both promising applications in health care and environmental cleanup and practical hurdles that need to be overcome before techniques that work in the laboratory can be made to work reliably in the real world.

In Chapter 5, Eric Tomlinson, of GENEMEDICINE, INC. (one of many new companies in the emerging biotechnology industry) provides an overview of the potential applications of biotechnology in health care. He suggests that, of all the new technologies, the most significant is the ability to manipulate the building blocks of life itself: to add or remove genes from cells and to transplant genes from one organism to another.

Savio L. C. Woo of Baylor College of Medicine focuses on the implications of this ability to manipulate genes for the treatment of disease, known as gene therapy. In Chapter 6, Woo clearly explains how gene therapy works (how genes are manipulated, packaged, and delivered to the patient) and what clinical effects the therapy has had to date.

Although gene therapy was originally conceived as a way to treat diseases that are wholly genetic in origin (such as hemophilia), Woo argues that it has potentially far wider applications, for example, in the treatment of cancer, infectious diseases such as hepatitis and acquired immune deficiency syndrome, cardiovascular diseases, and perhaps even neurodegenerative diseases such as Alzheimer disease.

Robert Nerem of the Georgia Institute of Technology describes the potential of biotechnology to develop bioartificial skin, cartilage, blood, and whole organs such as the pancreas and the liver. Pointing out that the need for tissues and organs for transplants far outstrips the supply available from donors, Nerem suggests in Chapter 7 that these techniques, which are collectively referred to as tissue engineering, may offer a solution to this perennial problem.

In Chapter 8, Michael Shuler of Cornell University analyzes the practical difficulties involved in manufacturing biotechnological products on a commercial scale. Living cells are complex organisms that often respond to subtle environmental changes in unpredictable ways, he argues, which can make it difficult not only to control product quality but also to predict how a product will behave when administered to a human subject.

Both Nerem and Shuler stress the need for an engineering-systems approach to solving such problems. Shuler urges the use of mathematical models to enable bioengineers to maximize a system's potential, thus improving production efficiency and lowering costs.

Shifting the focus from health care to the environment, in Chapter 9 Gene Parkin of the University of Iowa discusses bioremediation, the use of living organisms such as bacteria to destroy pollutants. This technology made headlines when it was used in Prince William Sound, Alaska, to ameliorate some of the environmental damage caused by the Exxon *Valdez* oil spill. Parkin explains the processes involved in bioremediation and examines some of the problems that must be solved for the technology to become a viable way of cleaning up environmental damage.

5

Effect of the New Biologies on Health Care

ERIC TOMLINSON

Human health care is being affected by the new biologies, particularly by the products that are emerging from the classical pharmaceutical industry and the new biotechnology industry. The pharmaceutical industry has global sales in excess of $200 billion per annum. The biotechnology industry, which had zero sales 5 to 6 years ago, now has sales of about $6 billion per annum. The goal of the biotechnology industry is to capture the remaining market by producing superior and effective products.

Today we are witnessing the advent of protein therapeutics and the ability to understand protein structure. We can look at the structure of DNA itself. We know that when DNA expresses a gene product it has to bend and that there are certain proteins present inside the nucleus that cause that bending to occur. Without such bending of DNA, the overall expression would be totally inefficient. We are also able to observe the structure of cells. We know that when macromolecules go into cells, they are recognized at the cell surface and go through defined pathways. Interaction of a ligand with a surface receptor results in many different types of trafficking events taking place within a cell.

We now know at the structural molecular level, not just at the phenomenological level, much of what happens within the cell in terms of cell processing, including knowledge about the secretion events that occur after a gene product is expressed. The pharmaceutical and biotechnology industries are exploiting this knowledge to try to gain access to target cells, be it for proteins or genes or biologically active RNA.

TABLE 5-1   Advances in Molecular and Cell Biology

Recombinant DNA and hybridoma technologies
Control of gene expression
Gene amplification (polymerase chain reaction)
Embryo stem cell manipulation
Efficient gene transfer
Protein and carbohydrate engineering
Instrumental analysis

What are these advances in molecular cell biology and how are these affecting the biotechnology industry? Table 5-1 lists some of the new advances that have been made. When the history of this era is written, the ability to manipulate mammalian embryonic stem cells, of all of these, will be seen to have been the most important of all. We are able now to go into a cell, alter its genetic makeup, and control cell differentiation. This step, first taken perhaps 20 years ago, produced events such as shown in Figure 5-1. This figure shows the development of two 11-day-old rat embryos. The embryo on the left is nondifferentiated because the gene for the growth hormone was removed. There was some differentiation, but then the growth stopped. When the gene coding for growth hormone was

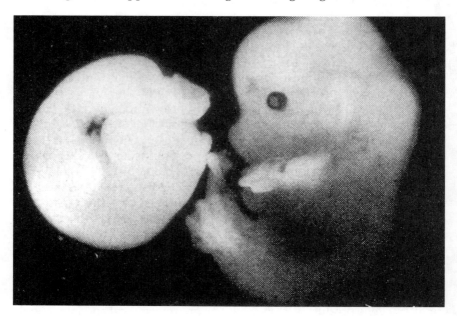

FIGURE 5-1   Two 11-day-old rat embryos. The embryo on the left is nondifferentiated.

Modern Medicines

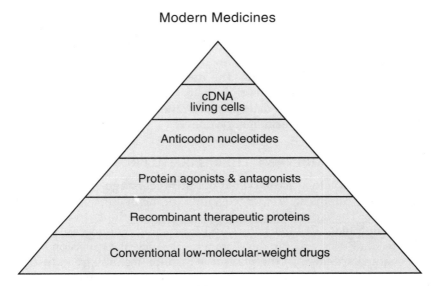

FIGURE 5-2   The development of the modern pharmaceutical-biotechnology industry.

returned to the embryonic cells, the embryo developed normally, as shown on the right.

This has given rise to hope, expectation, concern, and interest as well to the development of gene therapy and of so-called gene doctors. In 1985 *Business Week* devoted a cover story to this topic. The article stated that "hereditary diseases may soon be cured by manipulating human genes." Since 1985 we have seen the appearance of companies, such as my own and 40 other gene therapy companies worldwide, that are not just looking at genetic disorders to be treated with genes, but also at treating acquired disorders caused by environmental factors or a combination of environmental and genetic factors.

What is the effect of all these new biologies on human health care and particularly on health care products? Disease itself is now being understood, diagnosed, and treated at an increasingly higher order of genetic structure, function, and regulation. This means we are getting closer to understanding and controlling gene function within the body. Most drugs act directly or indirectly on gene expression. Antisense molecules affect gene function and gene structure, and the use of genes themselves as drugs is soon to be with us.

The development of the modern pharmaceutical-biotechnology industry in terms of modern medicines is shown in Figure 5-2. We all are aware of conventional low-molecular-weight drugs, such as aspirin or acetaminophen, which were discovered by trial and error or by serendipity. Recombinant therapeutic proteins were developed over the past 15 years. The newer developments include so-called targeted drugs, which are based on protein structure and are the low-molecular-weight agonists or antagonists of those proteins. The development of anticodon nucleotides, such as antisense and triple helix-forming DNA, and now the development of cDNA as a drug and even the use of living cells are part of the physician's future armamentarium.

RECOMBINANT THERAPEUTIC PROTEINS

The first protein was marketed about 6 years ago. Many different recombinant proteins have emerged, either for therapeutic or for diagnostic purposes. These developments resulted from an ability to understand how to manipulate DNA structure and expression. Polymerase chain reaction technologies and the development of efficient expression vectors have enabled scientists in the pharmaceutical-biotechnology industry to obtain high yields of protein from bacteria and now perhaps from plants. The creation of transgenic animals enables us to recreate human disease in animals so that we can efficiently and effectively study a putative drug product.

We are now successfully treating disease with therapeutic proteins. We have an adequate treatment for adult Gaucher's disease, which is an enzyme storage deficiency. The liver accumulates substrates and does not have the enzyme that can break down those substrates. Glucocerebrosidase, initially prepared by extraction rather than recombinant procedures, has alleviated this disease.

Myoscint, an antimyosin cardiac imaging agent, is a diagnostic agent that is based on proteins. When myocardial infarction occurs, the heart muscles rip open and myosin is exposed for the first time to the blood compartment and to an antimyosin antibody. Such an antibody, tagged with a gamma emitter, is administered intravenously and accumulates at the physical point of the infarction, where it can be detected by gamma scintigraphy during or just after myocardial infarction. This product has been followed by many new in vivo diagnostic imaging agents that are enabling the correct diagnosis and effective treatment of many different disorders.

PROTEIN AGONISTS AND ANTAGONISTS

Modern drug design involves designing a drug to fit a specific protein that is expressed by a specific gene. A protein structure may then be simulated on the basis of x-ray crystallography and, via computer, drug

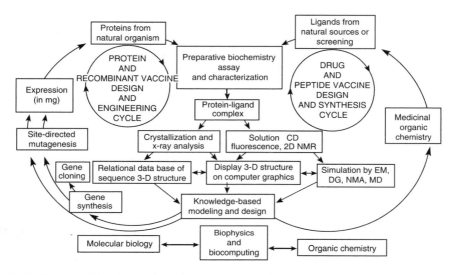

FIGURE 5-3 The design bicycle showing the flow of activities needed within the pharmaceutical-biotechnology industry to develop protein agonist and antagonist low-molecular-weight drugs.

molecules that could fit an active site in this protein are added to the structure. This process, combined with the advent of modern combinatorial chemistries, is dramatically changing the pharmaceutical industry's way of discovering drugs. Figure 5-3 shows the so-called design bicycle, which describes the flow of activities needed within the pharmaceutical-biotechnology industry to develop such protein agonist and antagonist low-molecular-weight drugs. The cycles are based on protein design and engineering and on drug design and synthesis and are a model for how the industry is restructuring itself (Blundell et al., 1990).

ANTICODON NUCLEOTIDES

The concept that RNA function, or even DNA function, can be inhibited by a complementary strand of RNA or DNA (antisense therapy) resulted from our improving ability to map the structure and function of the human genome, to understand better gene function and structure, to analyze disease at the genetic level, and to create transgenic animals and cells. The paradigm is that DNA is transcribed into messenger RNA and then translated into a protein. If that protein is an aberrant protein, as often occurs inside a tumor mass for example, then one can block the function of its messenger RNA by administering an antisense molecule that is complementary in its structure to the messenger RNA. This interaction then blocks the production of the aberrant protein. Clinical trials focusing on various molecular and disease targets are underway, largely brought about by the smaller biotechnology companies.

GENE THERAPY

The developments in the use of genetic material itself and living cells containing genetic material as therapeutic modalities have resulted from our ability to efficiently transfer genes into cells. Homogenous recombination is a very fertile research area, and the ability to harvest and to control the quality of cells has greatly enhanced our ability to consider living cells as therapeutic modalities.

Initial gene therapy programs in the late 1980s and early 1990s attempted to treat genetic disease. We tried to understand errors in genetic function and then how to correct that by using a gene as a therapeutic modality. However, most diseases are caused by both an environmental factor as well as by a genetic factor. Very few diseases are purely genetic in their origin, for example, Tay-Sachs disease and to some extent cystic fibrosis. Cholera and botulism are examples of diseases caused only by environmental factors. However, most diseases that will debilitate us as we get older and from which we will eventually die are caused by a polygenetic predisposition to disease that is affected by environmental factors. For example, some of us are predisposed to rheumatoid arthritis; environmental factors such as cold or damp weather will affect the inflammatory response and the development of this disease. Cancer is another example where there may well be a polygenetic predisposition that is sparked by some environmental factor. The gene therapy industry is beginning to think that perhaps there are a whole suite of diseases and clinical indications within each disease that can be treated using genes as therapeutics.

The advent of gene therapy was sparked off by the case of the "bubble boy," David, a 5-year-old boy who had severe compromised immunodeficiency disease (he lacked the enzyme adenosine deaminase). David had to live in a plastic chamber (a bubble) to remain impervious to adventitious viruses, which his immune system could not tackle. Unfortunately, he died before gene therapy was able to help him. Some years later the first human clinical trial in gene therapy took place in a girl named Amy Harper. Her white blood cells were taken from her body, the gene that codes for adenosine deaminase was introduced into those cells, and the cells were returned to Amy, who is alive and well more than 4 years later.

The method of putting the gene into Amy Harper's blood cells, which has now been used with many other patients with different clinical indications, was based on modifying a retrovirus. Harmful viral genes are removed and replaced with a useful gene, such as the gene coding for adenosine deaminase. The virus then infects cells, and healthy protein rather than harmful virus is produced, which is the rationale behind retroviral mediated ex vivo gene therapy. We were involved in developing a genetically altered skin patch. The skin patch is transduced by using retroviruses to contain a gene coding for growth hormone. This patch is layered onto normal skin and can produce and deliver its healthy proteins into the body of the patient.

Viral gene delivery systems are based on the fact that viruses effectively transfer genes into humans. The human cold virus, adenovirus, enters human fibroblast cytoplasm through a coated pit in the fibroblast surface. People have tried to use adenovirus to transfer human genes into patients. There are safety concerns about the use of defective viruses for gene therapy. What is emerging is the use of plasmid DNA for gene therapy. These are circular pieces of DNA derived from bacteria. Several companies, including our own, are inserting a therapeutic gene into a plasmid and then administering this genetic software as a pharmaceutical. Plasmid DNA can enter the nucleus but does not become integrated into chromosomal DNA; it remains episomal, or extrachromosomal (Figure 5-4). The administered therapeutic gene is transcribed into its messenger RNA, which is then translated into a therapeutic protein. The protein can be secreted from the cell to have an endocrine effect, such as insulin,

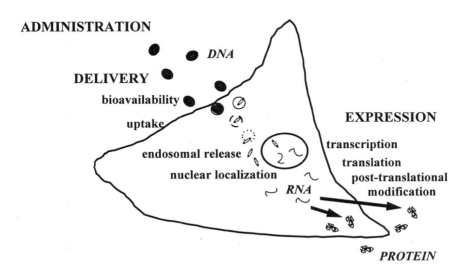

FIGURE 5-4   The use of a plasmid (administered DNA vector) as a pharmaceutical.

factor VIII, or factor IX; it can remain within the cell to have an autocrine effect and become a structural protein; for example it can be a receptor for low-density lipoprotein and assist in treating hypolipidemia; or it can actually leave a cell and then work in a paracrine fashion on neighboring cells, such as for a growth factor. The surface of the plasmid gene expression systems can be altered so that the system can target a particular cell. Numerous research groups are looking at placing sugars onto the surface of the plasmid that can recognize sugar receptors on cells. The use of plasmid-based gene expression systems coupled with advanced gene delivery methods is expected to be the next wave in gene therapy.

Gene therapy evokes a variety of concerns in people. All new and interesting areas of require a lot of scientific endeavor as well as a relationship among scientists, clinicians, regulatory bodies, and, of course, reimbursement agencies and patients for this type of treatment to be successfully introduced. Protein therapy had to go through the same process.

PRESCRIPTION FOR THE FUTURE

There is a long way to go: we still do not fully understand gene function nor do we know the structure of all genes and their controlling elements. Nonetheless, there is a driving force toward trying to develop drugs or modalities that control gene function and gene expression. Excellent scholarship in molecular and cell biology is taking place worldwide. A remarkable feature in the United States is the ability of scientists and others to commercialize that scholarship, to understand how that science can be developed into products. Scientists lend their names to biotechnology and pharmaceutical companies and can own part of the process—the American dream—and the American dream is now having a good effect on human health care. Advances are occurring in human health care because of that process.

TABLE 5-2   Therapeutic Protein Classes

Monoclonal antibodies
Interferons
Anticoagulants and thrombolytics
Colony stimulating factors
Dismutases
Erythropoetin
Human growth hormone
Interleukins
Tumor necrosis factor
Vaccines

A listing of the leading classes of therapeutic proteins shows that most product activity is still focused on cardiovascular diseases, diseases of the alimentary tract, antibiotics, and antibacterials (Table 5-2). The central nervous system remains as the next key target, with the problem of delivery of molecules as yet unresolved. Perhaps gene medicines will be the prescription for the future.

REFERENCES

Blundell, T. L., M. S. Johnson, J. P. Overington, and A. Sali. 1990. Knowledge-based protein modelling and the design of novel molecules. Pp. 209-249 in Protein Design and the Development of New Therapeutics and Vaccines, J. B. Hook and G. Poste, eds. New York: Plenum Press.

Tomlinson, E. 1991. Impact of the modern biologies on the medical and pharmaceutical sciences, J. Pharm. Pharmacol. 44 (suppl. 1):147-159.

6

Gene Therapy:
Beyond Genetic Diseases

SAVIO L. C. WOO

G ene therapy has three principal components. The first component is the therapeutic genes themselves. The gene discovery program, however, is not really within the domain of gene therapy. Therapeutic genes will continue to be discovered by investigators studying genes of interest to them. The discovery of new therapeutic genes will also result from the Human Genome Project. Thousands of human genes will be isolated, each with the potential to be a therapeutic gene. Dozens of human genes with therapeutic potential are already known.

Gene therapy refers to the development of science and technology for the delivery of therapeutic genes into the human body. This is the second principal component of gene therapy: how do we deliver the therapeutic genes to the proper organs with specificity, efficacy, and safety? This is the primary focus of gene therapy research today.

If we accomplish these goals, where will we go in the future? Once we can deliver a gene to a particular organ, we will want it to be expressed at a therapeutic level. The next step will be to regulate the expression of these genes. This is the third principal component of gene therapy, which will be important in the future: the development of expression and regulation vectors.

EX VIVO STRATEGY

There are two paradigms for gene therapy. The first one, the ex vivo strategy, is very straightforward. I will use the liver as an example be-

72

cause I am interested in metabolic diseases and the liver is the organ that I study. As shown in Figure 6-1, a piece of the liver can be surgically removed from the patient and dispersed into single cells in culture. Using any sort of delivery vehicle, an appropriate therapeutic gene can be transduced into the cells, yielding genetically reconstituted cells that can be transplanted back into the patient. Because the cells were originally derived from the patient, this is autologous transplantation and there should be no immunological rejection of the graft by the host. This procedure was completed in laboratory mice, rats, rabbits, dogs, and nonhuman primates. Five human patients are now undergoing this procedure as part of Dr. James Wilson's treatment of familial hypercholesterolemia at the University of Pennsylvania.

We have contributed to the development of this technology. However, when working with "large animal" models such as dogs, a piece of the liver is dispersed into billions of cells. Because these cells are cultured at a few million cells per dish, we need thousands of tissue culture plates. After having performed a few of these complicated procedures, I realized that this type of gene therapy is not the best approach for postmitotic tissues requiring the delivery of therapeutic genes to billions of cells.

The approach will be useful, however, for tissues with stem cells. For example, a few cells can be removed from bone marrow, transduced, and

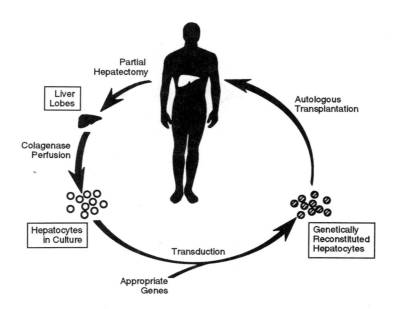

FIGURE 6-1   Ex vivo strategy for hepatic gene therapy.

then returned, and they will proliferate and take over a particular organ system. The ex vivo strategy will be very useful for this type of gene therapy.

IN VIVO STRATEGY

Future progress will need to be made on the second gene therapy paradigm, the in vivo strategy. With this strategy, therapeutic genes are delivered directly into the target organ, which is a far less complicated clinical procedure than the ex vivo strategy. The key element of in vivo gene therapy is the delivery vehicle. Three types of delivery vehicles are being explored: recombinant viruses, DNA protein complexes, and DNA liposomes. I will present data on the use of recombinant viruses as therapeutic gene delivery vehicles in living animal models.

USE OF RECOMBINANT VIRUSES: THE RETROVIRUS

The first recombinant virus used for gene therapy was the retrovirus originally developed by Dr. Richard Mulligan at the Massachusetts Institute of Technology. The retrovirus is a very simple RNA virus (Figure 6-2). It has two long-terminal-repeat (LTR) elements that control the expression of the viral genes. There is a packaging signal at one end and the viral

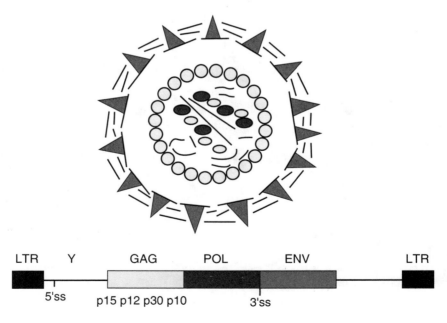

FIGURE 6-2 Retroviral structure. LTR; long terminal repeat.

genome is in the middle. There are only three viral genes coding for the core proteins, the envelope proteins, and the reverse transcriptase enzyme.

Dr. Mulligan removed all the viral genes and replaced them with a therapeutic gene, so that the recombinant virus contained the regulatory elements, the packaging signal, and a therapeutic gene. Using this recombinant virus, Dr. Mulligan demonstrated that the therapeutic gene can be transduced into a variety of cells in culture. The biology of the virus is such that when the cell is transduced, it incorporates the viral genome into the cellular chromosomes. The trait thus transferred becomes a permanent genetic trait of the cell; when the cell divides, the recombinant viral genome will divide with it.

One nice feature of this virus system is that because the transducing virus contains no viral genes, it is no longer capable of replication. Therefore, no continuous virus propagation occurs in the host, which is a very important concept in gene therapy.

Using this particular system, we treated a dog with a genetic deficiency in coagulation factor IX, which causes very severe hemophilia in animals. In normal dogs of this type, blood clots in about 8 to 10 minutes. In dogs with factor IX deficiency, blood clots in about 50 to 60 minutes. If these dogs were in the wild, they would all die from bleeding. A colony of these dogs has been well maintained and characterized at the University of North Carolina under the care of Dr. Kenneth Brinkhous. We collaborated with Dr. Brinkhous to try to deliver, via the retroviral vector, a canine factor IX gene to hemophilic dogs with the deficiency. The gene was delivered externally into a subcutaneous port implanted in the dog. The port was connected to a catheter inserted into the portal vasculature. Virus containing the therapeutic gene was infused slowly into this port, driven by a peristaltic pump. No anesthesia was given and our dog patient was wide awake. During the 1-hour procedure, the patient was on his four feet wagging his tail.

What were the results of this therapeutic procedure? The hemophilic dog began to make a small amount of clotting factor in the blood. The amount was very small, but the change in clotting time was dramatic. After gene therapy, clotting time was dramatically reduced from 50 to 60 minutes to 20 minutes (Figure 6-3). Expression of the therapeutic gene in this experiment lasted for 15 months, and the clotting time remained at 20 minutes.

This experiment shows that we can deliver genes to postmitotic tissue in which the cells have very long half-lives. In man, hepatocyte half-life is measured in years. We do not know how many years, but once we deliver the genes, they can continue to function and provide a therapeutic effect for a long time.

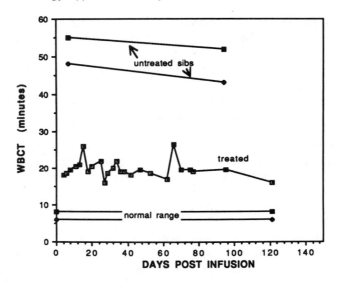

FIGURE 6-3   Whole-blood clotting times in a hemophilia B dog after retroviral-mediated hepatic gene transduction in vivo.

ADVANTAGES AND LIMITATIONS OF RETROVIRAL VECTORS

There are both advantages and limitations to using a retroviral vector for in vivo gene therapy. One advantage is that retroviral vectors have a very broad host-cell range, which enables the use of this therapy to treat a variety of diseases in different organs. This advantage is also a limitation, however, because it means that retroviruses lack tissue specificity and can only deliver therapeutic genes regionally, not systemically.

Another advantage is that the use of retroviral vectors results in permanent gene transduction, which potentially permits permanent gene therapy for genetic disorders. The limitation is that it transduces only dividing cells. In postmitotic tissues where the cells are not dividing, we have to stimulate the cells to divide before we can introduce the gene. Therefore, a surgical partial hepatectomy still had to be performed on our dog patient with hemophilia. Much research is currently under way on the use of chemicals to stimulate transient hepatocyte proliferation, so that the virus can be given to the liver cells without surgery.

This virus has an established safety record, at least for the ex vivo approach. Most of the approximately 50 approved clinical protocols of gene therapy in man use a retrovirus as the gene delivery vehicle. A limitation is that the virus has moderately low viral titer. If we have a preparation of recombinant virus at titers of 10^6 plaque-forming units (pfu)/mL, we consider it an excellent preparation. However, liver contains billions of hepatocytes and therapy will require many liters of this virus. Many laboratories are trying to increase the viral titer; success in this area can be expected in the near future.

ADENOVIRAL VECTORS

As we look at the advantages and limitations of retrovirus vectors, we need to be aware of the possibility of alternative factors for gene delivery that can provide the same advantages with fewer limitations. Adenovirus, a new vector used for gene therapy, normally infects the pulmonary epithelium and causes common colds, but it also has a very broad host-cell range in culture.

Shown in Figure 6-4 is a simplified genome map showing map units 0 to 100 for a 36-kilobase pair DNA virus. Investigators have replaced a segment of the viral genome with the therapeutic gene. This particular segment of the viral genome encodes a very important gene of the virus called E1A. This is, therefore, an E1A-deficient recombinant adenovirus. The E1A gene product is necessary for the expression of the rest of the viral genome. Without E1A the virus cannot replicate and thus can be used for gene delivery. This construct is conceptually very different from that of the retrovirus. In the retrovirus, all viral genes have been removed. In the adenovirus, all but one of the viral genes still remain in the vector.

What are the advantages of this vector? We took an adenoviral vector containing the β-galactosidase gene of *E. coli* and injected it directly into

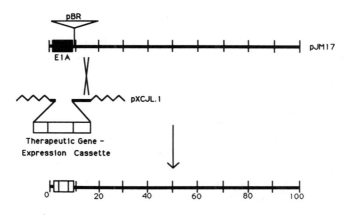

E1A⁻ Recombinant Adenovirus

FIGURE 6-4 Recombinant adenoviral vectors for gene therapy.

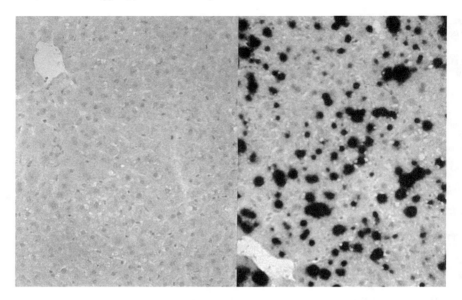

FIGURE 6-5 Mouse liver cells; blue indicates the presence of β-galactosidase. Left: mouse treated with control virus. Right: mouse treated with β-galactosidase gene.

the portal vasculature of laboratory mice without previous partial hepatectomy. We then sectioned the liver and stained it to look for blue cells that would indicate the presence of β-galactosidase. In the control mouse, given a control virus, shown on the left in Figure 6-5, there are no blue cells. In the mouse given the vector containing the β-galactosidase gene, shown on the right, about half the cells are blue. If we performed the same experiment with a retroviral vector, we would be lucky to see 1 percent blue cells. This vector, therefore, is extremely efficient for gene delivery, and its activity level as shown by enzymatic assay is tremendous.

Therefore, we made a recombinant adenovirus vector containing the canine factor IX gene and infused it into the portal vasculature of the hemophilic dogs. We measured the production of canine factor IX in the blood of the hemophilic animal (Figure 6-6). This is an antigen-negative model so there is no factor IX in the blood at time zero. Just 1 day after a single infusion of the virus, this hemophilic dog had accumulated 30 to 50 μg/mL of canine factor IX protein in the blood. The normal level of canine factor IX in an unaffected dog is about 10 μg/mL, so after one infusion of the therapeutic virus, this hemophilic dog was making 3 to 5 times the normal level of factor IX in the blood. Needless to say, after 1 day, the clotting time in this dog was normal. This example shows that using the adenovirus vector is a tremendously efficient method of gene delivery that can result in therapeutic levels of gene expression.

The problem is that after 1 week the level started to drop; in 3 weeks it dropped 100-fold. The curve then became biphasic; after 3 to 6 months the level returned to zero. So although this is a very efficient vector, it does not persist. Why not? It could be because the adenovirus is a lytic virus. Its business is to infect a cell, replicate, lyse the cell, and exit. It has no mechanism that enables it to persist in cells.

Another possibility is that these cells transduced by recombinant virus are expressing low levels of the viral proteins, even in the absence of E1A, and are being eliminated by the host's immune system. To determine whether this is the case, we performed the same experiment with another dog under immunosuppression.

The results were dramatic. Without immunosuppression there was a 100-fold loss of factor IX in 3 weeks. When we used cyclosporine A, the factor IX level persisted during the same period (Figure 6-7). These results suggest that the major contributing factor to the lack of persistence of the adenovirus delivery is viral antigen expression and subsequent elimination by the host's immune system.

It is therefore very important to think about the need to further modify the adenovirus vector backbone. If we could delete more viral genes so that the virus would no longer be able to express any viral function, what

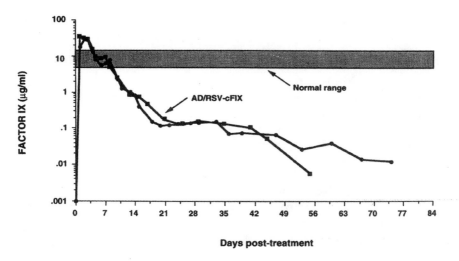

FIGURE 6-6 Plasma levels of canine factor IX in hemophilia B dogs after in vivo hepatic gene delivery.

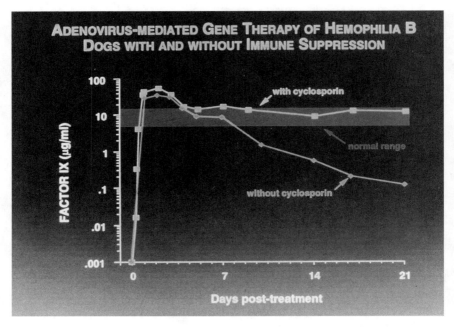

FIGURE 6-7   Bioassay after adenovirus injection with and without cyclosporine.

kind of persistence or duration of therapeutic period could we then achieve? The scientific community is working in this direction.

ADVANTAGES AND LIMITATIONS OF ADENOVIRAL VECTORS

The adenoviral vector for in vivo gene therapy has the advantage of very broad host-cell range, but it lacks tissue specificity. It is extremely efficient for gene transduction but lacks persistence. It transduces nondividing cells (with no surgery necessary) but it is a cytopathic virus.

When we did the experiment in the mice using the ß-galactosidase virus, we achieved 100 percent blue hepatocytes in vivo with a single shot, which is a remarkable result. If we increased the dose 5- or 10-fold, the animals died before our eyes. So this is a cytopathic virus, which presents the problem of overdosing. Overdosing is nothing new in medicine; every medicine, including aspirin, is toxic in overdose. This demonstrates the importance of considering the safety of vector systems for gene delivery.

Another advantage of the adenoviral vector is that it has very high viral titer. When we isolate these vectors they are in the range of 10^{11} pfu/

mL, 10^5 higher than the retrovirus. All we need is a few milliliters of viral solution: one shot in the arm and it's done.

We are trying to further engineer the adenovirus to give it persistence and to reduce cytopathicity. However, the development of this second-generation vector is going to take some time.

GENE THERAPY FOR SOLID TUMORS

We are now considering treating solid tumors with gene therapy. The adenovirus vector is desirable because we want to deliver therapeutic genes to a lot of cancer cells. Because the purpose is to deliver toxic genes into the cancer cells to kill them, it does not matter if the effect is transient. Toxicity also does not matter, because we want to kill the cancer cells anyway.

Kenneth Culver reported a couple of years ago that a *Herpes simplex* virus thymidine kinase (*ADV-tk*) gene was delivered into rat gliomas. Glioma cells had been injected stereotaxically into a hemisphere in the rat brain; the tumor cells had proliferated and grown into small tumors a few days later. (Such tumors continue to grow and eventually the animal dies from the brain tumor.) A retroviral vector containing the *ADV-tk* gene was introduced into the tumor directly by sterotaxic injection. The animals were then treated with either buffer or ganciclovir. Animals treated with buffer continued to grow large tumors and died. Tumors in animals treated with ganciclovir regressed.

I wanted to do the same experiment with the adenoviral vector. I thought that the limitations of the retrovirus vector could be offset with our adenoviral vector. The retrovirus is very inefficient with very low titers, which is why Culver did not use the retrovirus to cure the tumor and instead injected virus-producing mouse cells so that there would be enough virus production in vivo to treat the tumor.

Eight patients are now in clinical trials using that particular protocol, which is to inject virus-producing mouse cells into the tumor of human brain. That is a very inefficient process, and we think we can enhance the efficiency of gene delivery with the adenoviral vector.

In the original report, the authors argued that using a retrovirus is desirable for this type of gene therapy because biologically it transduces only dividing cells. It would only deliver the killer gene to the rapidly dividing tumor cells but not to the normal surrounding cells, thus providing a margin of safety. How do we deal with this if we use adenovirus? Ganciclovir by itself is not cytopathic. It diffuses in and out of cells just like any nucleoside, but if it diffuses into a cell that contains *ADV-tk*, it will be phosphorylated to become ganciclovir phosphate, which is a nucleotide. The nucleotide will then be incorporated into DNA in the dividing cells during DNA replication, causing chain termination that will lead to cell death. Thus, the mechanism of ganciclovir toxicity is also targeted for dividing cells, which makes the additional safety margin provided by the retrovirus redundant.

USING THE ADENOVIRAL VECTOR TO DESTROY TUMOR CELLS

With this in mind, we created an adenoviral vector containing the *ADV-tk* gene and used it in a glioma mouse model in mice. We injected the tumor cells into the brain and after 20 days the tumor grew to a large size. The results are shown in Figure 6-8: on the left is a mouse with a huge brain tumor. If we had waited for another day or two, this animal would have died. On the right is a mouse after gene therapy, and there is no evidence of a brain tumor. In Figure 6-9 we see on the top left the tumor that we resected from the brain. The tumor is about one-third the size of the entire brain. On the right is the brain after gene therapy; it looks perfectly normal and there is no evidence of tumor. There is a small black spot on the left hemisphere caused by our injecting the virus with a little charcoal to mark the site of injection. This brain shows no anatomic evidence of tumor.

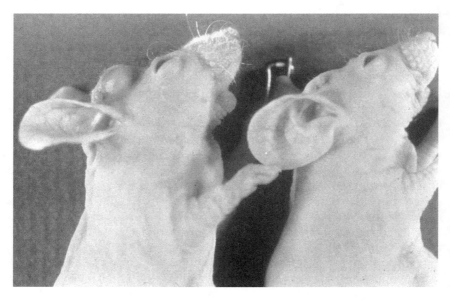

FIGURE 6-8   Gliomal mouse model in mice. Left: mouse with a large brain tumor. Right: mouse after gene therapy.

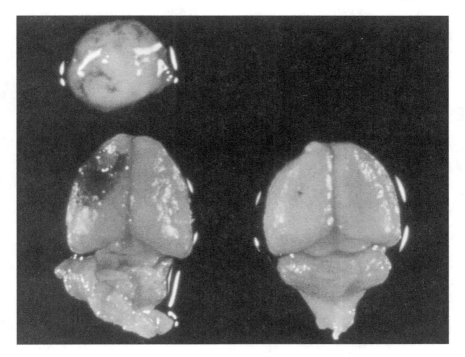

FIGURE 6-9   Brains from mice from gene-therapy experiment. Left: tumor (top) and brain from untreated mouse. Right: brain from mouse that received gene therapy.

What about pathologic evidence? Shown in Figure 6-10A is the brain from the animal treated with *ADV-tk* virus and given buffer afterwards. The tumor grew to enormous proportions, filling the entire hemisphere. It grew so big that it squeezed the rest of the brain and the ventricles actually disappeared. Figure 6-10B is a high-power section that shows an aggressively growing tumor that looks nothing like a normal brain. When the same experiment was done with animals treated with ganciclovir, the ventricles appear and there is no evidence of tumor (Figure 6-10C). The charcoal that was used to mark the site of injection can be seen under higher magnification (Figure 6-10D). This section looks like a normal brain with neurons, but there may still be a few residual cells that look like tumor cells. In some animals there is no evidence at all of residual tumor (Figure 6-10E, F).

We designed an experiment to provide quantitative data. We injected a large number of mice with tumor cells, divided the animals into two groups, and injected one group with a control virus, the other with a

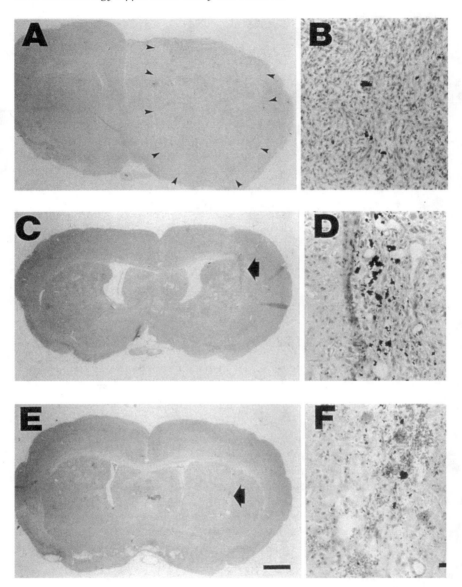

FIGURE 6-10   A, B: Growth of brain tumor treated with *ADV/tk* plus buffer; C, D: regression of brain tumor in mice treated with *ADV/tk* plus ganciclovir; and E, F: ablation of brain tumor in mice treated with *ADV/tk* plus ganciclovir.

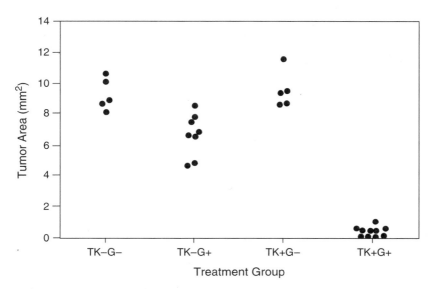

FIGURE 6-11   *ADV-tk* gene therapy for C6 gliomas in nude mice.

therapeutic virus. We then subdivided them into two smaller groups: one was treated with buffer, the other with ganciclovir. After 20 days (before the animals would have died if they had not had gene therapy) we killed all the animals, looked at the brains, and measured the tumor sizes.

Each point in Figure 6-11 represents one animal. The animals that received the control virus and no ganciclovir grew huge tumors. The animals that received the control virus with ganciclovir had much smaller tumors, which means that ganciclovir somewhat retarded the growth of the tumor but did not cause tumor regression. The animals treated with the therapeutic virus but no ganciclovir developed big tumors. The animals treated with the therapeutic virus and ganciclovir all had tumor regression. There were no exceptions. The results show the power of this technology in delivering killer genes to tumor cells to treat solid tumors.

CRITERIA FOR GENE THERAPY FOR BRAIN TUMORS

With these results, Baylor College of Medicine is preparing to propose a clinical trial using adenoviral-mediated gene therapy for brain tumors. As we look into the future, what are the criteria for using this gene therapy? In our view, the first criterion is that the tumor has to be a primary tumor or there has to be only limited metastasis, because the technology at this time involves injection of the therapeutic genes directly into the solid tumor. The second and third criteria are that the tumor must be accessible for injection and it must be nonresectable. The final criterion is that the patient must have a very poor prognosis with no possible alternative treatment. Brain tumors qualify for the trial because, more often than not, they satisfy all four criteria. Many gliomas are very aggressive and are not treatable by alternative methods.

What are our goals? There could be three: first, a long-term cure. If we can achieve that, we will all celebrate. Second, short-term regression would have tremendous value for the patients and their families. Third, palliation, which would improve the quality of patients' lives.

FUTURE OF GENE THERAPY

As we continue to look at gene therapy for cancer, are we going to stop at the brain? Can it be more generally applied? If you think about it, this is a virus that we can use to deliver genes into any solid tumors. The effect of ganciclovir is the same in all kinds of cells and it is not tumor specific. Therefore, why not think of other tumors as well? Indeed, Baylor College of Medicine has initiated an extensive program of gene therapy for solid tumors that includes many clinical investigators who collaborate with us. We are now working on tumors in the head and neck, colon, prostate, bladder, breast, and skin, among others. We have preliminary results for the head and neck tumors and for colon metastases in the liver.

What will gene therapy have in store for us in the future? What are the future challenges? Gene therapy started out to be a godsend technology for the cure of genetic diseases. It began with the first human trial under Dr. French Anderson. I have already talked about hemophilia. In cystic fibrosis, clinical trials are ongoing. As I have shown here, gene therapy for genetic disorders has really blossomed. We have developed technologies to deliver therapeutic genes to complement a genetic deficiency in living animals; will we be able to use the same technology to deliver killer genes to get rid of activities we do not want?

We are now entering into the era of gene therapy for acquired diseases such as cancer. Why should we stop with cancer? We should think about infectious diseases, such as acquired immune deficiency syndrome and hepatitis. All we need to do is to kill cells that are infected by the virus. What about cardiovascular diseases, such as atherosclerosis? At Baylor College of Medicine we have a program project supported by the National Heart, Lung, and Blood Institute on gene therapy for cardiovascular disease. In this particular project, we deliver the low-density lipoprotein receptor gene to laboratory rabbits. We have observed a dramatic reduction of serum cholesterol in these animals.

In the future the ultimate challenge will be for us to treat neurological diseases. It would be tremendously exciting to figure out what kind of therapeutic genes we could use to combat Alzheimer disease. Gene therapy feasibility demonstrations will be ample in the 1990s. We envision that gene therapy will have a major effect on medicine and health early in the twenty-first century.

ACKNOWLEDGMENT

Mark Kay conducted the hemophiliac gene-therapy experiments, which were supported by NIDDK grant 44080. Gretchen Darlington, Milton Finegold, and Mary Brandt are participating faculty and the collaborators at the University of North Carolina, Chapel Hill, are Dr. Kenneth Brinkhous and his collaborators. I would like to acknowledge my collaborators on the brain tumor project, particularly Dr. David Shine and Dr. Robert Grossman in the Department of Neurosurgery and Dr. Clay Goodman in the Pathology Department at Baylor. Dr. Shu-Hsia Chen, a postdoctoral fellow, performed the study in my lab.

7

Tissue Engineering: The Union of Biology and Engineering

ROBERT M. NEREM

Tissue engineering is an emerging part of biotechnology (Langer and Vacanti, 1993; Nerem and Sambanis, 1995). Biotechnology was defined by the Office of Technology Assessment a decade ago as techniques that use living organisms to make or modify products, improve plants or animals, and develop microorganisms for specific purposes. This definition emphasizes making or modifying a product by using living organisms and related types of activities.

The biotechnology industry, for the most part, might be called the genetic engineering industry, an industry based on recombinant DNA technology. Certainly this is an industry that makes products by using living organisms, usually genetically modified living organisms. There is also what I call the tissue-engineering industry; this industry also uses living organisms (i.e., living cells) and thus comes under the heading of biotechnology. This is an area that will become extremely important as we move into the twenty-first century.

A basic goal of tissue engineering is to fabricate living tissue equivalents, that is, biological substitutes to be implanted into the body. Also important is the development of materials that promote the remodeling of tissue or the resurfacing of a nonbiologic material to make it more compatible with the body. A critical issue is the growing of three-dimensional cellular structures. It is quite easy to grow cells in two dimensions in the laboratory but not so easy to grow cells in the three-dimensional structures that are important for any kind of tissue-engineered construct. Tissue engineering is also involved in developing vehicles for introducing genetically manipulated cells into the body (i.e., gene therapy).

Three things have to occur in tissue engineering. First, it is critical to understand the structure-function relationships. Second, cellular activity and function can then be controlled in collections of cells that have been assembled into tissues or organs, not only individual single cells. Third, once the ability to control exists, biological substitutes can be developed.

Understanding living organisms at the system level is all important in tissue engineering. Systems include the collection of cells and associated materials that make up the tissue and, ultimately, entire organs.

APPLICATIONS OF TISSUE ENGINEERING

Some applications of tissue engineering are artificial skin, bioartificial organs, blood substitutes, neurological implants, tissue-engineered vascular grafts, and various orthopedic devices (Langer and Vacanti, 1993; Nerem and Sambanis, 1995). An example of the last is tissue-engineered cartilage, which is being developed commercially.

One basic formula for tissue engineering involves taking cultured cells and putting them together with a supporting material. This material could be wholly synthetic or synthetic with an extracellular matrix of the normal adhesive proteins that are involved in the extracellular environment of the cells. When necessary nutrients are included, this becomes a living tissue equivalent. Environmental cues—the signals to which a cell is exposed—also influence living tissue. We now know that these signals are extremely varied and complex. From my perspective in mechanical engineering, I know that the mechanical environment of the cells is as important as the chemical environment, particularly for certain types of tissue and organs. Cells from these tissues and organs are extremely talented; they integrate the totality of their environment, including the mechanical stresses that they sense and that stimulate them.

To build biological substitutes, certain critical questions have to be answered. Should human cells be used? Should cell lines be used? Should cells be genetically modified? Are the cells going to express proteins at the level required for a particular tissue or organ? How are the cells going to respond to physiological stimuli? Will function be maintained long term? Will the materials used be biocompatible? Will the materials be stable long term?

ARTIFICIAL SKIN PRODUCTS

The Food and Drug Administration (FDA) has not yet approved a tissue-engineered product, but several products, particularly in the area of artificial skin, are in clinical trials and undoubtedly will be approved soon. Skin is a relatively simple tissue, and different approaches have been used to produce it (Bell et al., 1991; Coorper et al., 1991; Green et al., 1979; Yannas, 1992). One involves fibroblasts seeded in a collagen gel. Another uses fibroblasts seeded on a biodegradable material that provides a scaffold for cellular growth. A Boston company does large-scale expansion of epithelial cells, for example, taking a small amount of tissue from someone with extensive burns and expanding that cellular population to a size necessary cover the burned area. There also are acellular approaches in which materials and an extracellular matrix are used to promote wound healing and cellular growth.

Another example of artificial skin is skin equivalents that are used for toxicity testing. Models of this type are needed to test various products, such as cosmetics, for their toxicity. Having an artificial skin substitute reduces the number of animal experiments required to prove a product before commercialization.

BIOARTIFICIAL ORGANS

An important area for tissue engineering is the development of bio-artifical organs. These may be of a hybrid nature, involving synthetic materials together with living cells and other natural components.

At the Georgia Institute of Technology (Georgia Tech), one of the tissue-engineering projects, directed by Dr. Thanassis Sambanis, is to develop a bioartificial pancreas as an approach for treating insulin-dependent diabetes. This alternative to insulin injection or other forms of treatment is being pursued in several laboratories and involves the implantation of insulin-secreting cells to create an artificial pancreas with living pancreatic cells that are responsive to glucose and secrete insulin (Colton and Avgoustinatos, 1991; Reach, 1993; Tziampazis and Sambanis, 1994). Immunoprotection or immunoisolation is achieved by encapsulating the cells in a membrane-like biomaterial. The feasibility of using such implants with exogeneic cells to treat diabetes mellitus has been demonstrated in both small and large animal models (Lanza et al., 1991, 1993). Human trials are now underway (Soon-Shiong et al., 1994).

A key question is cell availability. Isolation of the primary beta cells from animal glands is difficult. Primary eyelets cannot be amplified in culture, but it is possible to engineer glucose-responsive, insulin-secreting cell lines, and this is being done. A line that has been used at Georgia Tech is the βTC3 line, but we plan to use the better lines that are now available (Efrat et al., 1988). Regarding the use of native cells or genetically manipulated cells, we think that engineered cell lines should be used for the bioartificial pancreas.

Figure 7-1 is an illustration of such an encapsulated bioartificial pancreas. This is the system being used at Georgia Tech (Tziampazis and

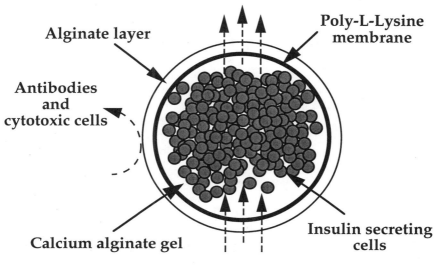

Insulin and metabolites out

Alginate layer

Poly-L-Lysine membrane

Antibodies and cytotoxic cells

Calcium alginate gel

Insulin secreting cells

Glucose, nutrients in

FIGURE 7-1 Illustration of immunoisolated insulin-secreting cells or spheroids in alginate/poly-L-lysine/alginate polymer, provided by the courtesy of A. Sambanis.

Sambanis, 1995). It has either cells or spheroids of cells inside the membrane, which has a molecular-weight cutoff that provides immuno-isolation. The membrane permits insulin to be secreted and the cells inside to sense the glucose environment and thus be responsive to glucose.

Researchers at Brown University have been using encapsulated cells for cell therapy for nervous system disorders (Bellamkonda and Aebischer, 1994; Tresco et al., 1992). As an example of a technique for physically targeting the delivery of biologically active molecules, this could be considered to be a form of drug delivery.

Another important application of tissue engineering is the development of a bioartificial liver. I have been a scientific advisor to a group in Minneapolis that is working on this. It is a joint project between the University of Minnesota and a company named Regenerex. This project is important because although 2,500 liver transplants are performed in the United States each year, 27,000 patients go without organ replacement and some die while on the waiting list. In the future a goal would be the development of an artifical liver that involves long-term hepatocyte culture (Dunn et al., 1991). However, in the short term the focus of many efforts is the development of a bridge-to-transplant system.

One such system being developed in Minneapolis uses a hollow-fiber bioreactor in which hepatocytes reside (Shatford et al, 1992). The blood is removed from the patient; passed through this system, where it become detoxified; and then perfused back into the body. The cells are inoculated with collagen, which then polymerizes, and the collagen contracts to form a collagen gel within the hollow fibers in which cells reside. Within the hollow fibers, there is a lumen stream that provides for nutrients and waste-product removal. The blood passes over the hollow fibers around the outside. Experiments have been done with small animals, but applying this technology to humans involves considering the issue of scale-up.

Obviously, applying such a system to a human requires a considerable increase in the number of cells used. Experiments now use rat hepatocytes; should a different species be used in humans? Should the flow characteristics of the bioreactor be different for humans? As the system is scaled-up, many things change, including the hydrodynamic environment, mixing characteristics, and nutrient delivery. These issues are important in developing such a extracorporeal, bioartificial liver system as a bridge to transplant.

VASCULAR SYSTEM

My own interests have focused on the application of engineering to the vascular system. Much of the research in my laboratory has been in the area of heart disease and the influence of blood flow on vascular biology and the processes that are important in the development of the initial stages of atherosclerosis. Progression of this disease in the coronary blood vessels results in myocardial ischemia, even in a heart attack. The surgical treatment involves bypass surgery, where areas of obstruction are bypassed by a saphenous vein or a mammary artery. Everyone is familiar with this procedure and knows people who have undergone bypass surgery.

We believe that the mechanical environment of a blood vessel is all important (Nerem, 1993). Basically, a blood vessel is a conduit for flowing blood. The blood has a pressure associated with it that acts as a mechanical force on the vessel wall. As blood flows over the vessel wall, it also imparts what we call a shear stress, which is a frictional force. Just as air moving over an automobile provides a frictional drag, blood flowing through a vessel provides a frictional force on the vessel wall. The approach of our laboratory at Georgia Tech is first to understand vascular biology; second to control cellular function within the context of a blood vessel; and third, through tissue engineering, to construct a blood vessel substitute. Throughout this process it is important to understand the role of mechanical forces (i.e., the mechanical environment in which the cells will reside).

Figure 7-2 shows the morphology of endothelial cells both in static culture and after exposure to a laminar flow and the associated shear stress for 24 hours (Levesque et al., 1989). The response to laminar flow is

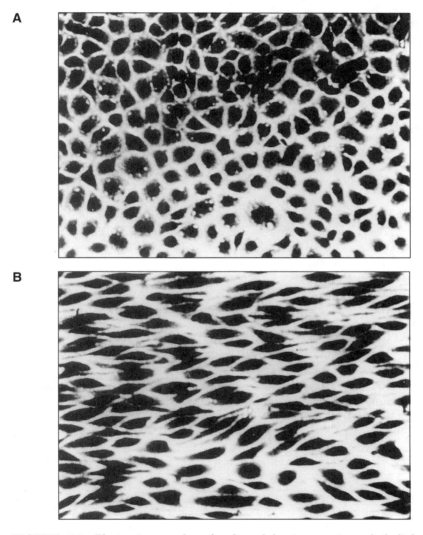

FIGURE 7-2 Photomicrographs of cultured bovine aortic endothelial cells grown under controlled conditions (A) and under shear stress (85 dynes/cm^2) for 24 hours (flow from right to left). Reprinted with permission from the American Society of Mechanical Engineers.

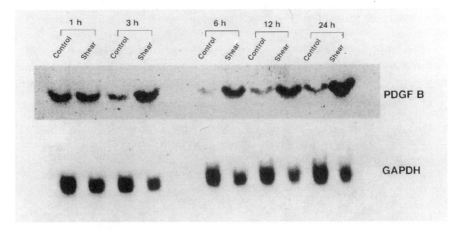

FIGURE 7-3 Flow stimulates platelet-derived growth factor messenger RNA expression in endothelial cells as shown by Northern blot analysis. Reprinted with permission of the American Physiological Society.

cell elongation and an alignment of the cell's major axis with the direction of flow. This response is active and involves a reorganization of the cell's cytoskeletal structure. An example of this is F-actin, a major structural component within the cell: microfilaments relocate from the dense peripheral band pattern characteristic of static culture to stress fiber bundles aligned with the direction of flow. This reorganization reflects itself in the mechanical properties of these cells. Thus, there is a major difference in morphology and structure associated with the mechanical environment imposed by the laminar flow. Endothelial cells exposed to flow are much more like what we see in vivo in animals and in human beings, except for regions of low flow or stasis.

Laminar flow also influences function, for example, the secretion of various biologically active molecules. This is illustrated in Figure 7-3, where a Northern blot for a particular molecule (platelet-derived growth factor B chain) is presented (Mitsumata et al., 1993). Messenger RNA levels are shown for a control experiment and a flow experiment at different times. Gene expression under control conditions and flow conditions changes significantly over time. Thus, the influence of mechanical forces extends to the level of gene expression. These mechanical forces are part of the environmental cues that regulate the expression of genes.

RECONSTITUTING BLOOD VESSELS

Unfortunately, some people do not have native vessels available for use in bypass surgery. Either they have had bypass surgery before or their vessels are not suitable. Thus, an important goal is to develop small-diameter vascular grafts for use in the coronary system. Various approaches have been taken, including the use of synthetic materials. In one approach, a synthetic material is seeded with endothelial cells, the cells that line blood vessels and provide the natural interface between flowing blood and the underlying vessel wall (Zilia et al., 1987). This hybrid vessel then becomes the vascular graft. There has been some initial success with this approach.

Others are pioneering what are called acellular approaches involving the implantation of a material that promotes cell ingrowth. Thus, although the endothelial cells have not been seeded on the material, over a relatively short period of time the cells grow in from neighboring regions of the vasculature.

In my laboratory we are very interested in reconstituting a blood vessel in culture (Ziegler and Nerem, 1994). This work builds on the work of Weinberg and Bell (1986). We are taking smooth muscle cells that constitute the vessel wall, endothelial cells that provide the inner lining, and appropriate extracellular matrix components and putting them together in the form of a blood vessel.

As a first step we are developing a model for our vascular biology experiments that we believe will be a much better simulation of the in vivo environment for cell culture studies (Zeigler et al., 1995). This model involves plating endothelial cells on top of a collagen gel in which smooth

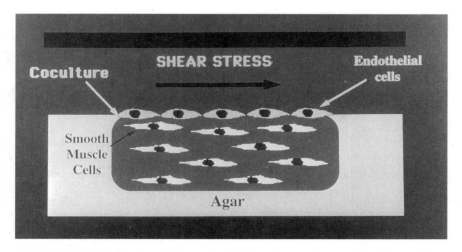

FIGURE 7-4 Illustration of the endothelial cell–smooth muscle cell co-culture model of the blood vessel wall being used in a laminar flow chamber at Georgia Tech.

muscle cells reside (Figure 7-4). We have just started experiments to look at the effects of flow on such a co-culture system. As we move toward tissue-engineered biological substitutes, it will be important to simulate the real physiologic environment as closely as possible in the cell culture laboratory. We believe that adding flow to the static culture models of vascular cells that have been used in the past is a step in the right direction. However, the endothelial cells inside your body do not reside on a plastic surface; they adhere to a basement membrane and have neighboring smooth muscle cells. In this new model we can look at mechanical force effects (flow effects) on endothelial cells along with their normal neighboring partners, the smooth muscle cells. We are in the process of extending this to a tubular configuration, and our long-term goal is to develop a vascular substitute for bypass surgery. Tissue engineering—whether it involves a blood vessel substitute or some other tissue or organ—requires a great deal of understanding of cell biology and molecular biology and an ability to put cells together as a system to develop tissues and organs.

NEW BIOMATERIALS

Biomaterials are an important core technology for tissue engineering (Peppas and Langer, 1994). Some people believe that for the past 25 years, biomaterials have been in their age of innocence. Much work has been done with good intentions, but maybe with a certain amount of naivete, at least in the sense of thinking there such a thing as a passive material. However, now we are in the age of discovery, in which materials are being developed that interact with cells and tissues specifically, where we can even build certain receptor-like sequences into the surface of the biomaterial to facilitate appropriate interaction (Massia and Hubbell, 1991).

Tissue engineering is bringing microfabrication and nanofabrication technology together with molecular and cell biology (in a combination that can be called the nanotechnology of life). Basically, we are taking nanotechnology in a normal engineering sense and bringing it together with "nano" biology. If we can learn how to bridge from microfabricated systems into cell behavior, including subcellular events, it will be possible to develop prostheses that are much more effectively coupled to a person's normal body. At the Georgia Tech Microelectronics Research Center, surfaces can be built where the scale of an electric field or a magnetic field is considerably less than that of a single cell. This provides the opportunity for an interaction between an electronic system and a cellular system at the single-cell level. There also is the possibility of incorporating controlled-release polymers for drug delivery at the nano scale. As useful as

such technologies will be in basic research, they have wide-ranging implications in the coupling of systems within the body to man-made devices.

CURRENT STATE OF TISSUE ENGINEERING

Most people think of biotechnology only as the genetic engineering
(i.e., recombinant DNA) industry. However, a tissue-engineering industry is emerging, an industry that is 10 to 15 years behind the classical
recombinant DNA technology industry, but one that still is an important
area for future development. In the United States each year there are
20,000 transplants but there are 2,000,000 implants. There are 100,000
people with transplants, but 10,000,000 people with implants. The need
for implantable parts and devices is staggering, and this need cannot be
met through organ and tissue transplantation. This is an enormous opportunity for the tissue-engineering industry. Today it is estimated that
the industry consists of approximately 20 companies with about 3,000
employees and $200 million in research and development expenditures.
Within a decade the total commercial sector dollar volume could easily
increase tenfold to $2-5 billion.

There are many other examples of the potential of tissue engineering:
work is being done with cartilage, with the expansion of bone marrow
stem cells, and in the field of neurology. It is an exciting area that in a
sense began with the biological revolution: the ability to culture cells
outside the body. This revolution led to many advances in cell and molecular biology and is an important foundation for tissue engineering.

How are tissue engineering and genetic engineering related? To start
with, cellular implants may involve cells that have been genetically manipulated. Also, tissue-engineered substitutes may be useful as vehicles
for introducing genetically modified cells. Because gene therapy can be
viewed as the most sophisticated form of tissue engineering, there is an
overlap between these two exciting areas. In building our tissue engineering program at the Georgia Institite of Technology in partnership with
Emory University School of Medicine, we have made gene therapy a
priority.

Another area of importance to tissue engineering is that of drug delivery, or more precisely, the delivery of biologically active molecules.
There are many reasons for targeting drug delivery, and many groups are
beginning to look at systems to do this (Langer, 1990). It would be advan-
tageous to deliver drugs specifically to an organ or a tissue. This would
give a therapeutic dose at the desired site while having a low systemic
dose in nontarget compartments. Such targeted delivery will not only
reduce the risk of side effects and tolerance effects, but also facilitate
combination drug therapies. Some delivery systems may involve the in-

teraction of receptor molecules characteristic of cells and of drugs or the physical aspects of delivery. Because delivery of drugs to the right site at the right dose is important, not drug efficacy in the petri dish, a delivery system should not be an afterthought. Engineering the design of the drug and its delivery system should be concurrent.

There has been a cultural revolution in this country in terms of the importance of biology; I think we need a further cultural revolution in terms of the role of engineering in biology. Engineers need to be involved not only on the production side, but also very early in the research and development process, as they are in other areas of science and engineering. How a product is manufactured depends on how the product was developed and thus is based on scientific investigation. Engineers need to be involved across the entire spectrum of activity from basic research all the way to the final product. Only then will one have a seamless commercialization process.

I also think there is going to be yet another cultural revolution. As we learn more and more about biology from an engineering perspective, as we learn how biological systems have been engineered for us, the use of engineering to develop products for nonbiological, nonmedical applications will radically change. Thus, as we move into the twenty-first century, not only is there a role for engineering in biology with all the resulting applications, but biology has the potential for enormously altering engineering.

REFERENCES

Bell, E., M. Rosenberg, P. Kemp, R. Gay, G. D. Green, N. Muthukumaran, and C. Nolte. 1991. Recipes for reconstituting skin. J. Biomech. Eng. 113:113-119.

Bellamkonda, R., and P. Aebischer. 1994. Review: tissue engineering in the nervous system. Biotechnol. Bioeng. 43:543-554.

Colton, C. K., and E. S. Avgoustinatos. 1991. Bioengineering in development of the hybrid artificial pancreas. J. Biomech. Eng. 113:152-170.

Cooper, M. L., J. F. Hansbrough, R. L. Spielvogel, R. Cohen, R. L. Bartel, and G. Naughton. 1991. In vivo optimization of a living dermal substitute employing cultured human fibroblasts on a biodegradable polyglycolic acid or polyglactin mesh. Biomaterials 12:243-249.

Dunn, J. C. Y., R. G. Tompkins, and M. L. Yarmush. 1991. Long-term *in vitro* function of adult hepatocytes in a collagen sandwich configuration. Biotechnol. Prog. 7:237-245.

Efrat, S., S. Linde, H. Kofod, D. Spector, M. Delannoy, S. Grant, D. Hanahan, and S. Baekkeskov. 1988. Beta-cell lines derived from transgenic mice expressing a hybrid insulin gene-oncogene. Proc. Natl. Acad. Sci. USA 85:9037-9041.

Green, H., O. Kehinde, and J. Thomas. 1979. Growth of cultured human epidermal cells into multiple epithelia suitable for grafting. Proc. Natl. Acad. Sci. U.S.A. 76:5665-5668.

Langer, R. 1990. New methods of drug delivery. Science 248:1527-1533.

Langer, R. and J. P. Vacanti. 1993. Tissue engineering. Science 260:920-926.

Lanza, R. P., D. H. Butler, K. M. Borland, J. E. Staruk, D. L. Faustman, B. A. Solomon, T. E. Muller, R. G. Rupp, T. Maki, A. P. Monaco, and W. L. Chick. 1991. Xenotransplantation of canine, bovine, and porcine islets in diabetic rats without immunosuppression. Proc. Natl. Acad. Sci. U.S.A. 88:11100-11104.

Lanza, R. P., P. Lodge, K. M. Borland, M. Carretta, S. J. Sullivan, A. M. Beyer, T. E. Muller, B. A. Solomon, T. Maki, A. P. Monaco, and W. L. Chick. 1993. Transplantation of islet allografts using a diffusion-based biohybrid artificial pancreas: long-term studies in diabetic, pancreatectomized dogs. Transplant. Proc. 25:978-980.

Levesque, M. J., E. A. Sprague, C. J. Schwartz, and R. M. Nerem. 1989. The influence of shear stress on cultured vascular endothelial cells: the stress response of an anchorage-dependant mammalian cell. Biotechnol. Prog. 5:1-8.

Massia, S. P. and J. A. Hubbell. 1991. Human endothelial cell interactions with surface-coupled adhesion peptides on a nonadhesive glass substrate and two polymeric biomaterials. J. Biomed. Mater. Res. 25:223-242.

Mitsumata, M., R. S. Fishel, R. M. Nerem, R. W. Alexander, and B. C. Berk. 1993. Fluid shear stress stimulates platelet-derived growth factor expression in endothelial cells. Am. J. Physiol. 265:H3-H8.

Nerem, R. M. 1993. Hemodynamics and the vascular endothelium. J. Biomech. Eng. 115:510-514.

Nerem, R. M., and A. Sambanis. 1995. Tissue engineering: from biology to biological substitutes. Tissue Eng. 1(1):3-13.

Peppas, N. A., and R. Langer. 1994. New challenges in biomaterials. Science 263:1715-1720.

Reach, G. 1993. Bioartificial pancreas. Diabetic Med. 10:105-109.

Shatford, R. A., S. L. Nyberg, S. J. Meier, J. G. White, W. D. Payne, W.-S. Hu, and F. B. Cerra. 1992. Hepatocyte function in a hollow fiber bioreactor: a potential bioartificial liver. J. Surg. Res. 53:549-551.

Soon-Shiong, P., R. E. Heintz, N. Merideth, Q. X. Yao, Z. Yao, T. Zheng, M. Murphy, M. K. Moloney, M. Schmehl, M. Harris, R. Mendez, and P. A. Sandford. 1994. Insulin independence in a type I diabetic patient after encapsulated islet transplantation. Lancet 343:950-951.

Tresco, P. A., S. R. Winn, and P. Aebischer. 1992. Polymer encapsulated neurotransmitter secreting cells. Potential treatment for Parkinson's disease. ASAIO Trans. 38:17-23.

Tziampazis, E., and A. Sambanis. 1995. Tissue engineering of a bioartificial pancreas: modeling the cell environment and device function. Biotechnol. Prog. 11:115-126.

Weinberg, C. B., and E. Bell. 1986. A blood vessel model constructed from collagen and cultured vascular cells. Science 231:397-399.

Yannas, I. V. 1992. Tissue regeneration by use of collagen-glycosaminoglycan copolymers. Clin. Mater. 9:179-187.

Ziegler, T., R. W. Alexander, and R. M. Nerem. 1995. An endothelial cell–smooth muscle cell co-culture model for use in the investigation of flow effects on vascular biology. Ann. Biomed. Eng. 23:216-225.

Ziegler, T., and R. M. Nerem. 1994. Tissue engineering a blood vessel: regulation of vascular biology by mechanical stresses. J. Cell. Biochem. 56:204-209.

Zilia, P. P., R. D. Fasol, and M. Deutsch, eds. 1987. Endothelialization of vascular grafts. Basel: Karger.

8

Development of Biopharmaceuticals: An Engineering Perspective

MICHAEL SHULER

J urassic Park, the book and the movie, exposed millions of people to a vision of life in a biotechnology company. The company portrayed in the film was a commercial failure for many reasons. The brilliant molecular biologist worked with DNA in a rather abstract manner, without knowing and without wanting to know much about the biology of the organisms involved. The project failed because the components, not the system, were optimized and because secrecy demands made it so that no timely outside advice was obtained from uninvolved experts.

The question we will explore is: Could some of these factors, in this fiction, affect real-life biopharmaceutical firms? This presentation is from an engineering perspective, a perspective that is often missing in the decision-making process of many biopharmaceutical firms. It is missing in part because engineers and their employers have defined the role of engineering too narrowly. Engineering has been defined in terms of skill rather than in terms of systems, and a systems perspective is the key to making a product efficiently and, even more importantly, to knowing if a product will have value.

An engineer sees a living cell as a complex chemical plant. It has its own regulatory system and has many built-in redundancies for safety. A living cell has a far more sophisticated control system than has ever been put into a chemical plant designed by humans.

I will begin here with a discussion of therapeutic proteins, the products that have made the biopharmaceutical industry successful, and then discuss other products that are emerging, products dependent on and independent of DNA knowledge. Finally, I will consider recent trends in terms of their implications for education.

THERAPEUTIC PROTEINS

Simple strategies based on simple linear logic were initially conceived for the development of therapeutic proteins: a gene plus its expression produced a protein, which in turn produced a product system. The logic behind its use was that the product would attack the disease and this would lead to health improvement. This strategy, however, can fail. If you want to make protein, and just make protein, you are in the soybean business. If you want to sell a pharmaceutical product, you must worry about protein quality and biological activity. Is the protein correctly folded? Are appropriate sugars added? Are there multiple species present?

When biotechnology first began, many people thought that simple bacteria or yeast could make all proteins. They did not realize that these organisms lack some of the key processing steps needed for the necessary product quality, at least for some of the protein products. These initial processes were often problematic, in many cases because each component was optimized separately without any thought given to the integration of the components.

The situation has changed a lot over the past 15 years. Much has been learned: projects are developed with integrated teams, multiple host systems are explored, and the choice of the host system is closely linked to product quality. The issue of product quality, however, has not been fully resolved. Product quality is a function of culture conditions and, potentially, of the scale-up conditions used to make it.

Post-Translational Processing

We are familiar with the language of DNA in terms of nucleotides: how they are put together, how that information is transcribed into RNA, and how RNA is translated into proteins (Armstrong, 1989). Proteins are described as linear sequences; post-translational events include folding, glycosylation (putting on sugars), disulfide bond formation (which is dependent on redox potential), and phosphorylation, all of which are dependent on the physiological environment. In addition, protein are sometimes altered (clipped off) during transport or secretion.

Correct post-translational processing is often key to the therapeutic value of the product (Bialy, 1987; Liu, 1992). Will it have the right immunogenic characteristics? Will it be targeted to the right tissue? Will the body clear it before it has a chance to have a therapeutic effect? Correct post-translational processing depends on the intrinsic capabilities of the cell, which are determined by genetics and culture conditions (Monica et al., 1993).

The physiologic utility of antibodies can depend on how they were produced (Van Brunt, 1990). Immunoglobulin M (IgM) produced in mice in ascites fluid has a half-life of 780 minutes. IgM can be also be produced in cell culture. Mouse cells can be used to make hybridomas that are hybrids of slow-growing, antibody-producing lymphocytes and fast-growing myeloma (cancer) cells. Hybridomas in serum-free medium in an air-lift reactor (a reactor in which air circulates and oxygenates the culture) can produce IgM with a half-life in the body of only 3 minutes, which is not long enough for therapeutic use. The same hybridoma cells in medium containing a small amount of serum in a hollow-fiber reactor, which may protect cells from shear, produce IgM with a half-life of 18 minutes. This range of half-life from 3 to 780 minutes demonstrates the sensitivity of the use of the product to variations in production.

Use of Mammalian Cells

Bacteria were found to be incapable of performing glycosylation. Yeast can do some simple glycosylation, but not the complex glycosylation that occurs in humans, and yeast have a bad habit of going wild and continuing to add sugars (Hodgson, 1993). The insect cell baculovirus system (Luckow, 1991) is of interest, but it is unclear if that system can produce the complex glycosylation reactions found in mammalian systems. Consequently, many products are now made by mammalian cell cultures.

Chinese hamster ovary cells are used in many cell cultures. These cell cultures are very expensive and difficult to use but have been brought into full commercial production. Their use was approved by the Food and Drug Administration (FDA) despite initial reservations about safety (Ramabhadvan, 1987). These cells are transformed cells; they are immortal and will continue to divide forever. Because all cancer cells are transformed cells, there was some concern about the possibility that a product produced by Chinese hamster cells would induce cancer in humans. Consequently, there are very severe regulatory constraints on the mononucleic acids, for example, that can be present in one of these products.

There also was concern about using mammalian cells because of the presence of endogenous viruses and about using viral vectors that were disabled viruses of primates because of the possibility of their reverting to virulence. Such problems did not occur, but for a long time there was much resistance to using these cells.

Use of the Chinese hamster cells results in a good yield of product, but it takes a long time to achieve the yield. This system is much slower than many other systems, and because the yield is often compromised, this is a very expensive way to produce proteins (Hodgson, 1993).

Problems with Scale-Up

It is impossible to duplicate the conditions in a small reactor when scaling up to a large reactor. Shear and mixing time will be different and the cells will be in a somewhat different environment in the large-scale reactor (Shuler and Kargi, 1992). Potentially a biopharmaceutical firm might conduct Phase I clinical trials with a product that was developed on a modest scale and end up unintentionally conducting larger-scale trials with a different product. The difference would result from the subtle changes in post-translational processing due to heterogeneities in the large-scale system that alter cell physiology. We do not know how to predict when this is going to occur, and a great deal of fundamental work is needed in this area. Often we do not have full control of the quality of the product we are making when we go to a larger scale.

Even if we can make the identical product at the larger scale, we still sometimes face problems in recovery and purification. Many of the steps in recovery and purification can alter side groups on the proteins, which increases the number of different forms of the protein that are present in the product. The extent to which post-translational processing affects the therapeutic value of a protein is unclear, but in many cases we know it is important. This is an issue that the FDA has not fully resolved. The primary hurdle remaining in the production of therapeutic proteins is the issue of product quality control.

SMALL MOLECULES

The era of therapeutic proteins being used in vaccines is drawing to a close. Therapeutic proteins will still be important products for many years and new products will be developed, but proteins are very awkward to use as therapeutics. As we become more sophisticated in our knowledge, there will be more emphasis on the use of small molecules.

Our knowledge of DNA can be used as the basis for making small molecules via metabolic, or pathway, engineering (Bailey, 1991). We can insert into a cell a gene that will encode an enzyme. That enzyme can augment the flux of material down a particular metabolic pathway or it can be used to generate totally new pathways. It is clear that if we do this there is a problem of optimization. If I send 100 percent of the material down one particular pathway, the rest of the cell, the rest of the infrastructure, would collapse. It is also clear that sending zero down the pathway does not make any product. So there is an optimum between those two options that has to be designed.

People have tried to apply metabolic control theory to get a better sense of the optimal conditions. However, in many such applications, people have not adequately taken into account that the product of a particular pathway may affect, directly or indirectly, the material that feeds into the pathway. These applications have only looked at part of the cell and not the whole cell.

There are some good examples where metabolic engineering may prove fruitful. Polykeytide antibiotics and anticancer agents have been produced from *Streptomyces* (McDaniel et al., 1993). Through this route, we can generate many novel structures that may lead to compounds that will be of significant medicinal use.

Biotechnology has led to ways of designing compounds via chemical synthesis of, for example, oligonucleotides and nucleotide analogs. Antisense technology is based on the production of oligonucleotides. These will be areas in which biopharmaceutical firms will be involved.

Carbohydrate drugs seem poised to enter the market. These tend to mimic some of the sugars that are added to proteins. In many cases, sugars are what is recognized by a receptor protein in the signaling process, and a carbohydrate component could be used to mediate physiological functions. Cell adhesion molecules are being investigated because they have been involved in cancer metastasis, arthritis, and other medically important conditions.

EPIGENESIS

The products discussed so far are based on DNA knowledge. This knowledge presumes a model where unique genes have unique effects on physiology. That is a paradigm that has worked well in diseases such as hemophilia and has served the biopharmaceutical industry well. However, this paradigm can fail and the concept of genetic determinism can fail.

Ninety-eight percent of diseases have a strong epigenetic factor. The rules governing cellular and physiological regulation are located not in the chromosome, but in the complex interactive nonlinear metabolic networks resulting from multiple gene expression. These epigenetic networks organize cellular and physiological responses to environmental signals (Strohman, 1994). Biopharmaceutical firms must understand the limitations that epigenetic networks can place on the success of single gene products and on gene therapy. For many polygenic complex disorders, such as cancer, the epigenetic network will ultimately control an individual's fate; a single gene will not always control response.

The p53 Gene

We know about the p53 gene and how its mutation is linked to cancer. An analogy can be made with the two-brake car used for driver education. The p53 gene is the brake that we can put on cell proliferation. For example, a mouse has been constructed in which both p53 alleles are absent, which means that both brakes are missing. You might expect in such a circumstance that the driver education car (the mouse) would crash. Yet, in these experiments the mice were all normal at birth and early developmental growth was normal. In adulthood many of the mice developed cancer far in excess of the control population, but there were still some mice that never developed cancer. Why? Because there was an emergency brake. Other gene products, and in some sense the whole epigenetic network, were able to functionally replace the p53 gene product. There is a great deal of redundancy built into biological systems. Thus, genetic analysis showing a mutation in the p53 gene in a single allele in a single cell does not mean that cancer will develop. So there is a distinction between being able to determine predisposition and being able to predict what will happen. This situation is similar to that of the car with only an emergency brake, where there potentially is a higher probability of a crash than when both brakes are working.

The epigenetic system, however, is often neglected in discussions about the results of the Human Genome Project. When you work with bioprocesses, you have to deal with epigenetic responses. When a normal p53 gene is introduced into a p53-defective cell, it may or may not restore normal growth regulation. It depends on the type of mutation that has occurred in the p53 gene. So a biopharmaceutical firm that embarks blindly on making a p53 product can certainly not be guaranteed success.

Effect of Environment

Another way of looking at this is that many genotypes can give rise to a single phenotypic functional form. The same genotype can give rise to different phenotypes in different environments. Thus, genes are necessary but not necessarily sufficient to determine outcomes. Epigenetic behavior means that the history of the organism becomes important: previous as well as current environments are important.

When you build a bioprocess, you need to be careful how you prepare your inoculum. It has to be done in precisely the same manner every time if you want the same results. The same is true when you treat disease. You have to realize that the patients, even with the same genes, may not be the same if they have been exposed to different environments.

When we encounter very complex interactive systems, it is often important to have mathematical models to help us consider those systems. Such models can help us ask "what if" questions, identify knowledge gaps, and test alternative mechanisms. They probably can help us to reasonably predict what is going to happen with a large population, although in terms of any individual the predictions are probably not valid.

It is surprising and somewhat disconcerting that the biological community as a whole barely tolerates mathematical models. About 12 years ago, I had one paper rejected by a microbiology journal—a paper in which I used a mathematical model—based on a reviewer's comment that the laws of thermodynamics did not apply to living systems.

There have been failures with biopharmaceutical products caused by an inability to predict how the products were going to interact with complex systems. Three companies met their Waterloo over sepsis products that had to work in a very complex ecology, not only within cells but with microorganisms involved in sepsis. The inability to predict interactions in complex systems was the principal reason clinical trials did not support the development of those products.

A nucleotide analog (fialuridine) that was given in a recent trial for hepatitis B at the National Institutes of Health (NIH) resulted in the deaths of 5 of the 15 patients (Cimons, 1993). There was unexpected inhibition of replication of liver mitochondria. Because it takes a while for mitochondria to be replaced, taking patients off the drug did not immediately alleviate symptoms.

Fialuridine had previously been given to patients with acquired immune deficiency syndrome (AIDS) but was withdrawn because it did not appear to have much therapeutic effect. At least three other nucleotide analogs are either being used on AIDS patients or are in clinical trials. Here again, the difficulty will be our inability to appreciate the interaction throughout the whole system.

BIOLOGICAL SYNTHESIS

The pharmaceutical industry is interested in switching from using chemical to using biological synthesis. When you make products via chemical synthesis, you often end up with right-handed and left-handed molecules. When you use these drugs, you hope that one enantiomer gives you the therapeutic effect and the other does nothing. Sometimes the other enantiomer causes adverse effects in patients. Because biological synthesis results in products with just one orientation (Stinson, 1993), we are going to see increasing emphasis in pharmaceutical firms on biotransformations using modulated cells or enzymatic synthesis.

DRUGS FROM PLANT PRODUCTS

We are also going to see many new drugs from natural products. These products are essentially empirical: we can get some clues about them from their use by primitive societies, which have accumulated a wealth of knowledge about which plants to use and when to harvest them. For example, if warm milk is used to extract the product, that tells you something about the nature of the product. There is tremendous untapped genetic diversity in plants, perhaps even more so in marine systems, particularly marine algae. I have seen estimates of 250,000 to 500,000 for the number of plant species. Many, of course, are disappearing very quickly, before they can be cataloged. Between 5,000 and 40,000 have been tested for pharmaceutical activity (Abelson, 1990; Svoboda, 1989). We have 120 prescription drugs worldwide that are based on extracted plant products. The question is, to what extent are we missing other opportunities?

Right now at least nine compounds from plants or marine algae are in preclinical trials for both AIDS and cancer (Anonymous, 1992). For pharmaceutical firms to pursue these kinds of products, there needs to be an enabling technology that ensures that this product can be made in quantities useful for testing and ultimately for production. So the supply issue becomes important.

Taxol: A Case Study

Much of the interest in natural products was renewed because of taxol, which comes from the bark of the Pacific yew tree. There was a good deal of publicity about it a few years ago, partially because it appeared to be a very exciting drug, the best anticancer drug that had come along in about 15 years. It has been approved for use against ovarian cancer and is in advanced clinical trials with breast and lung cancers. It is also in clinical trials against several other cancers. The ultimate therapy will probably be a combination therapy with cisplatin or some other chemotherapeutic drug. These clinical trials were greatly impeded because of the problem of taxol supply. Until this point the National Cancer Institute (NCI) had always presumed that if they needed a compound, it could be made in quantities sufficient to test it. This was not the case with taxol (Cragg et al., 1993).

Sam Broder, chief of NCI, said that taxol was the first but would not be the last product where the supply would be the critical issue. Why was the supply a critical issue with taxol? It comes from the bark of the Pacific yew tree. It takes about 18 months to dry the bark before it can be extracted to produce the product. It takes three 100-year-old trees to generate enough bark to treat one patient. (There is nothing magic about a 100-year-old tree, it just takes many more 2-year-old trees to supply enough bark.) Pacific yew trees are among the slowest growing trees in North America and are fairly uncommon. The Pacific yew is the home of the spotted owl, which caused much controversy with environmentalists. In a sense, environmentalists were pitted against cancer patients.

So there was a need to look for alternative supplies. The taxol molecule is very complex. Just recently it was announced that total synthesis has been achieved (Nicoleou et al., 1994; Holton et al., 1994a, b). However, the synthesis was achieved by a route that will never be commercially useful. The chemistry is still important; it gives us some clues in terms of taxol analogs that may be more easily administered or more effective than taxol.

Producing taxol by genetic engineering is very unlikely. Part of the problem is that NIH has funded a great deal of work on bacteria and on mammalian cells but very little fundamental work on plant cells. We know far less about the biochemistry, genetics, and physiology of plants than we do about *E. coli* or about mammalian cells. No one knows the pathway for taxol production or what enzymes are involved. We do not know where the genes are located or how they are regulated. So in the short term, genetic engineering is not a likely route for making a product such as taxol or other products from algae or plants.

Another route, however, is being commercially developed now. You can extract a precursor of taxol from common yews and convert that precursor into taxol by a semisynthetic method. Taxol can also be extracted directly from the needles of the ornamental yews, but this is probably not a promising route because of the complexity of the needle extract (e.g., pigment co-elutes with taxol).

Plant Cell Tissue Culture

The final possibility is plant cell tissue culture (Payne et al., 1992; Shuler, 1993). One of the advantages of plant cell tissue culture is that you can be assured of an expandable supply and the quality will be the same in June as it is in January, which is not true with natural plant material. With plant cell tissue culture it is possible to select high-yielding variants much more easily. The product can be much cleaner (fewer contaminants present) than a product from the natural extraction, either from needles or from bark. Finally, novel products can be generated in such systems, such as novel taxanes. The question will be whether such novel taxanes have any useful biological activity.

In my laboratory we have worked on plant cell tissue culture for about 20 years and have been fortunate to be supported by the National

Science Foundation (NSF). Our work has been directed toward enabling technology, and we have developed several strategies for producing secondary metabolites from plant cells (Payne et al., 1992). I believe that one important role for government funding is support of enabling technologies. The presence of such technologies makes possible the development of products that might otherwise be abandoned.

Two of my students formed a company that is taking the strategies we developed and trying to apply them to taxol. I am on the board of directors of this company but have no financial interest in it. For example, I am principle investigator of a consortium grant from NCI to Cornell University that involves another academic institution, two commercial companies (one of which is the one started by my students), and a government lab. We are trying to better understand the scientific basis of the production of taxol in tissue culture, but the mixture of private, academic, and government labortories generates many possibities for conflict of interest.

With a cell line developed by Ray Ketchum at the U.S. Department of Agriculture, we have been able to achieve at least 20 milligrams of taxol per liter. An article in *Science* reported a fungus that made taxol (Stierle et al., 1993). The level that we have achieved is nearly one million times higher than the level that was achieved in the fungus, which means that a one-liter reactor could make as much taxol as could a million-liter reactor with the fungus, assuming there were no other improvements in production.

We have also seen novel taxanes with some cell lines under some culture conditions. We have not yet had a chance to explore their bioactivity. These observations argue that plant cell culture of taxol is a plausible possibility. Commercial development of plant cell tissue culture is on track in meeting all of the milestones that have been set.

It has been very satisfying to see ideas that we worked on for 20 years being put into practice. My colleagues told me that it was not worth working on plant cell tissue culture because there was no commercial processing and there probably never would be; although there had been a commercial process of plant cell tissue culture in Japan, this had not been done in the United States. The support of NSF for the development of enabling technology was very important.

I find that even though I know the principals in one of the companies very well, there are sometimes awkward situations. I have to remember, for example, if I heard something while I was a member of the company board of directors or while I was the director of the RO1 NIH grant supporting educational research in the same general area. One is confidential, the other can be discussed freely.

Epigenetic Behavior of Plant Cell Culture

If you do not believe in epigenetic behavior, you should work with plant cell culture. There is one cell line we have that produces about 10 milligrams of taxol per liter. We have had it go through cycles where it produced, then it did not produce, then it produced, and then it did not produce again. The genetics had not changed, but cells are sensitive to history. If you have a certain procedure for how you subculture that cell line, you had better be very religious about following it. You had better use the same size flask, the same type of cap, the same level of inoculum: everything had better be the same. If you are going to work with these cell lines you have to very careful and very sensitive to the history of the culture as well as to the environmental cues that you are giving the culture.

IMPLICATIONS FOR EDUCATION

There are other upcoming products in biotechnology. We will be hearing a lot more about tissue engineering and gene therapy. There will be a market for biopharmaceutical firms to produce viral vectors to enhance gene therapy. There may be a market for customized products for treating cancer with a patient's own specific immunological markers. The biopharmaceutical industry will continue to change and its needs will affect our graduates.

Several trends are clear. One trend affecting every major industrial sector is that research and development growth is strongest in small companies. Small companies emphasize flexibility and are able to rapidly move to market. New health care economics will place greater emphasis on efficient production systems and on products with clear therapeutic advantages. Companies that can predict the product winners will succeed; companies unable to anticipate their product's effectiveness in complex systems may fail. Companies with inefficient processes will ultimately pay a stiff penalty.

In such an environment, graduates will be required to understand systems, either to predict effectiveness or to produce products efficiently. Graduates who are expert in a small subsystem but cannot realistically relate that subsystem to the whole process will become as extinct, perhaps, as Jurassic Park dinosaurs.

Finally, breadth will become increasingly important. A perspective from discovery to process to market and an understanding about product usefulness will be needed. However, students still must have depth in at least one subarea of biotechnology; depth cannot be sacrificed to breadth.

* * *

In *Jurassic Park*, John Hammond had a great vision and drove the project, but his vision blinded him to many of the dangers of the project. Henry Wu, who focused totally on the technical molecular level, simply had no vision at all. The advisory board was present, but they knew too little too late, and that may be a recipe for failure for any biopharmaceutical firm.

REFERENCES

Abelson, P. H. 1990. Medicine from plants. Science 247:513.

Anonymous. 1992. Natural product agents in development by the United States National Cancer Institute. J. Natural Prod. 55:1018-1019.

Armstrong, F. B. 1989. Biochemistry. 3rd ed. New York: Oxford University Press.

Bailey, J. E. 1991. Toward a science of metabolic engineering. Science 252 :1668-1675.

Bialy, H. 1987. Recombinant proteins: virtual authenticity. Bio/Technology 5:883-889.

Cimons, M. 1993. Experimental hepatitis drug proves deadly in clinical trial. Am. Soc. Microbiol. News 59:596-597.

Cragg, G. M., S. A. Schepartz, M. Suffness, and M. R. Grever. 1993. The taxol supply crisis. New NCI policies for handling the large-scale production of novel natural product anticancer and anti-HIV agents. J. Nat. Prod. 56:1657-1668.

Holton, R. A., H.-B. Kim, C. Somoza, F. Liang, R. J. Biediger, P. D. Boatman, M. Shindo, C. C. Smith, S. Kim, H. Nadizadeh, Y. Suzuki, C. Tao, P. Vu, S. Tang, P. Zhang, K. K. Murthi, L. N. Gentile, and J. H. Liu. 1994a. First total synthesis of taxol. 2. Completion of the C and D rings. J. Am. Chem. Soc. 116:1599-1600.

Holton, R. A., C. Somoza, H.-B. Kim, F. Liang, R. J. Biediger, P. D. Boatman, M. Shindo, C. C. Smith, S. Kim, H. Nadizadeh, Y. Suzuki, C. Tao, P. Vu, S. Tang, P. Zhang, K. K. Murthi, L. N. Gentile, and J. H. Liu. 1994b. First total synthesis of taxol. 1. Functionalization of the B ring and first total synthesis of taxol. J. Am. Chem. Soc. 116:1597-1598.

Hodgson, J. 1993. Expression systems: a user's guide. Bio/Technology 11:887-893.

Liu, D. T-Y. 1992. Glycoprotein pharmaceuticals: scientific and regulatory considerations, and the U.S. Orphan Drug Act. Trends Biotechnol. 10:114-120.

Luckow, V. A. 1991. Cloning and expression of heterologous genes in insect cells with baculovirus reactors. Pp, 97-152 in Recombinant DNA Technology and Applications. A. Prokop, R. K. Bajpai, and C. S. Ho, eds. New York: McGraw-Hill.

McDaniel, R., S. Ebert-Khosla, D. A. Hopwood, and C. Khosla. 1993. Engineered biosynthesis of novel polyketides. Science 262:1546-1551.

Monica, T. J., C. F. Goochee, and B. L. Maiorella. 1993. Comparative biochemical characterization of a human IgM produced in ascites and in vitro cell culture. Biotechnology 11:512-515.

Nicoleau, K. C., Z. Yang, J. J. Liu, H. Ueno, P. G. Nantermet, R. K. Guy, C. F. Clalborne, J. Renaud, E. A. Couladouros, K. Paulvannan, and E. J. Sorensen. 1994. Total synthesis of taxol. Nature 367:630-634.

Payne, G. F., V. Bringi, C. L. Prince, and M. L. Shuler. 1992. Plant Cell and Tissue Culture in Liquid Systems. New York: Hanser Publishers.

Ramabhadvan, T. V. 1987. Products from genetically engineered mammalian cells: benefits and risks. Trends Biotechnol. 5:175-179.

Shuler, M. L., and F. Kargi. 1992. Bioprocess Engineering: Basic Concepts. Englewood Cliffs, N.J.: Prentice-Hall.

Shuler, M. L. 1993. Plant cell culture: an approach to exploiting the genetic and chemical diversity of higher plants. Pp. 58-67 in Research Opportunities in Biomolecular Engineering: The Interface Between Chemical Engineering and Biology. Washington, D.C.: U.S. Department of Health and Human Services.

Stierle, A., G. Strobel, and D. Stierle. 1993. Taxol and taxane production by *Taxomyces andreanae*, an endophytic fungus of Pacific yew. Science 260:214-216.

Strohman, R.1994. Epigenesis: the missing beat in biotechnology? Biotechnology 12:156-164.

Stinson, S. C. 1993. Chiral drugs. Chem. Eng. News Sept. 27:38-65.

Svoboda, G. H. 1989. Society news. Am. Soc. Pharmacol. Newslett. 25(2):6.

VanBrunt, J. 1990. The importance of glycoform heterogeneity. Biotechnology 8:995.

9

Bioremediation: A Promising Technology

GENE F. PARKIN

In this country over the past 20 to 30 years, we have contaminated our environment with a wide variety of organic and inorganic chemicals. Environmental professionals have been given the charge of cleaning up this environmental contamination, with the general goal of protecting the public health. Bioremediation is one of the emerging technologies that environmental professionals use to attempt to remedy these contamination problems. The objective of this chapter is to discuss bioremediation: to describe how it works, its advantages and limitations, and what we need to know to better apply the technology in the future.

Bioremediation is generally considered to be an emerging technology. Most environmental professionals feel that bioremediation is an attractive alternative, because it offers significant potential for cost-effective, environmentally acceptable treatment of contaminated waters and soils. However, no treatment technology is a panacea, applicable to all situations. This is reasonably well documented in a 1993 report from the National Research Council's Committee on In Situ Bioremediation, which states:

> Bioremediation offers significant potential for cost-effective, environmentally acceptable treatment of contaminated waters and soils. However, bioremediation is clouded by controversy over what it does and how well it works, partly because it relies on microorganisms, which cannot be seen, and partly because it has become attractive for "snake oil salesmen" who claim to be able to solve all types of contamination problems. As long as the controversy remains, the full potential of this technology cannot be realized.

113

The report describes the technology as having some controversy and confusion associated with it. One of the major objectives here is to attempt to remove some of this controversy, to give an idea of when we might apply bioremediation and what we need to know to successfully apply it in the future.

We can start with a general definition of bioremediation as the use of living organisms, or the catalysts that they produce, to bring about the removal or destruction of pollutants that contaminate a wide variety of substances, such as water, wastewater, and soils. We have even applied biological processes to contaminated gas streams. The major focus here will be the use of bacteria in bringing about bioremediation, but other organisms, such as fungi, plants, protozoa, and algae, are also used to facilitate bioremediation.

AN EMERGING BUT NOT A NEW TECHNOLOGY

Bioremediation is an emerging technology, but we need to recognize that it is not really a new technology. Environmental engineers (in the past we were called sanitary engineers) have been using biological processes to solve various contamination problems for at least a century, using processes such as anaerobic digestion for treating sludges from wastewater treatment plants in the 1880s, trickling-filter treatment of domestic wastewater in 1894, activated-sludge treatment of domestic wastewater in 1914, and biological treatment of industrial waste waters in the 1930s. Over 20 years ago (in 1972), the first documented success of in situ bioremediation was reported by Richard Raymond, who is thought by some to be the father of bioremediation. Thus, the use of biological processes to remove or treat pollution is not new, except for perhaps the name bioremediation.

The question then is, what is new? In my opinion, two things are new. First is the chemicals that we are trying to biodegrade: anthropogenic and so-called xenobiotic chemicals. Anthropogenic chemicals enter the environment primarily as a result of human activity; xenobiotic chemicals are "foreign" to natural biota. One might think of it as the difference between degrading something that is relatively degradable, such as sugar, and degrading a chlorinated solvent, such as trichloroethylene.

The second new aspect of the problem is the complexity of the medium or matrix that has become contaminated with these chemicals. Most of this discussion will focus on subsurface contamination—the contamination of our groundwater environment—because that is the area where bioremediation can dramatically affect our ability to cleanup these sites. However, these situations are extremely complex and present major engineering challenges.

THE UNDERGROUND ENVIRONMENT

We are interested in bioremediating three segments of the underground environment that can become contaminated: the near-surface soil (the vadose or unsaturated zone, which includes some moisture and some soil gas), the aquifer (the water), and the solid materials. These segments can become contaminated in numerous ways by numerous chemicals. As shown in Figure 9-1, a chemical in area A might be the spill of a light nonaqueous-phase liquid (LNAPL) such as gasoline, which will spread out over the groundwater table when it migrates down through the vadose zone because it is lighter than water. Then, of course, it will at least partially dissolve in the water and move with the groundwater flow, contaminating the water and the soil or the aquifer materials with which the water comes in contact (area B). Aquifers can also become contaminated with dense nonaqueous-phase liquids (DNAPLs), which have a density greater than water so that they sink to the bottom of the groundwater table (area C), dissolve, diffuse, and contaminate the aquifer (area D).

The complexity of cleaning the underground environment has been described by Perry McCarty (1994) of Stanford University as follows: take your hand and put it in a bucket of motor oil and make a fist, and then pull the fist back out of the motor oil. Now the job is to remove all the oil from your fist. You can repeatedly submerge your fist into buckets of clean water and you will remove some but not all the oil. You can submerge your fist into buckets of warm soapy water and remove more of the oil, but not all of the oil. You can blow hot air all over your hand, and maybe remove some additional oil, but you cannot remove all the oil

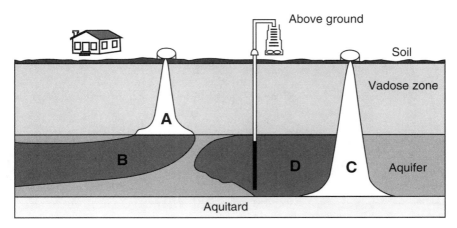

FIGURE 9-1   Treatment domains. Adapted from McCarty (1994).

without opening up the fist. Yet, that is our challenge. Bioremediation offers significant potential for attacking these problems.

EX SITU AND IN SITU BIOREMEDIATION

There are two general types of bioremediation. Ex situ, or above-ground bioremediation (Figure 9-1), involves the design, construction, and operation of an engineered reactor above the ground. Water is pumped out of the ground or soil is dug up, made into a slurry, and then put into a reactor that is located above the ground. Bioremediation in the ground is referred to as in situ bioremediation.

In situ bioremediation will be the major focus here, because this is where there is significant potential for improvement. In situ bioremediation can proceed in two ways. It can be natural (sometimes termed intrisinic bioremediation), which means no action is taken other than to monitor the site. The idea is that if the rate at which the microorganisms are degrading the pollutant is faster than the rate at which the pollutants are leaving the site, the site will cleanse itself. However, more often we are interested in engineered in situ bioremediation, in which materials are added to the ground to stimulate the growth of organisms. Nutrients such as nitrogen and phosphorus may be needed. An electron acceptor such as oxygen might be added. Trying to deliver these materials represents a significant engineering challenge, and may even include introducing microorganisms into the subsurface environment.

The scheme shown in Figure 9-2 demonstrates some of the general ways in which we might do this (MacDonald and Rittmann, 1993). Many

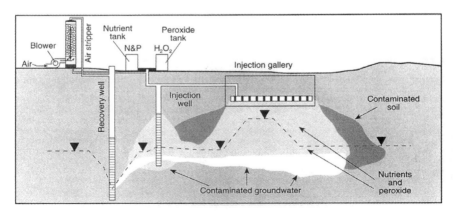

FIGURE 9-2 A system for treating regions above and below the water table. Reprinted with permission from MacDonald and Rittmann (1993).

modifications are possible. The dotted line represents the groundwater table, and contamination both above and below the water table is treated. For example, nitrogen and phosphorous might be added by using an injection well or in an infiltration gallery, which may simply be a perforated pipe in the ground. Groundwater would then be moved in one direction or another, perhaps by using an extraction well. As water and soil gas are removed via this extraction well, above-ground treatment could also be used. Treated groundwater can be reinjected, by using groundwater recirculation, to meet a target cleanup standard. In situ bioremediation involves adding materials to the ground, making sure that the microbes come in contact with all the materials that are necessary for organisms to grow. Obviously, if an anaerobic, or reduced, bioremediation scheme is desired, hydrogen peroxide as an oxygen source would not be added.

WHY BIOREMEDIATION?

A few statistics will indicate the potential for bioremediation. It has been estimated that more than 200 million tons of hazardous materials are generated in this country each year (Wentz, 1989), and more than 50,000 sites have been identified that need some type of remediation (Gibson and Saylor, 1992). It also has been estimated that 40 million people live within 4 miles of a Superfund site (Gibson and Saylor, 1992). Of the 2 million underground storage tanks that are storing only gasoline, as many as 600,000 are leaking or expected to leak soon (Bakst and Devine, 1993). Because 50 percent of the U.S. population gets drinking water from groundwater, this presents a potentially significant problem. The most recent estimates indicate that cleanup will cost around $1.7 trillion (Gibson and Saylor, 1992). Some are now estimating that bioremediation might be a $500 million per year industry by the year 2000 (MacDonald and Rittmen, 1993). So, there is tremendous potential for the application of bioremediation.

Why might we want to use bioremediation? What drives environmental professionals to want to use this process? Bioremediation is one of the few processes that can actually destroy pollutants, converting organic materials into carbon dioxide, water, chloride, and other minerals. Biological processes may cost less than physical and chemical processes. In situ bioremediation has additional, potentially important advantages over pump-and-treat technology (pump the water above ground to treat it). Because the organisms are grown near the pollutant, the process may occur more quickly. This is particularly important for hydrophobic compounds, which tend to "stick" to the soil material. If organisms are growing near where the hydrophobic compounds are adsorbed, the equilibrium between the liquid and the solid can be destroyed and the chemicals can begin to desorb from the solids and be biodegraded. If these processes are occurring in the ground, there is no need to dewater (remove water from) the aquifer.

LIMITATIONS

Remembering that no treatment process is a panacea, it is very important to understand the limitations of a given treatment technology, and there are limitations to the technology of bioremediation. First, it is not universally applicable. Because we are dealing with potentially toxic compounds, there is a danger that the organisms that you are trying to grow will be killed. Toxic intermediate compounds may be produced by these organisms. The classic example is anaerobic biotransformation of trichloroethylene into vinyl chloride, which is a known human carcinogen. Most people feel that vinyl chloride is more of a health problem then the parent compound. Finally, in situ chemical reactions or organism growth may clog wells or aquifers.

Figure 9-3 illustrates the feasibility of in situ bioremediation by plot-

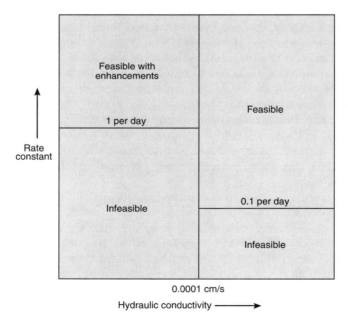

FIGURE 9-3 Feasibility of in situ bioremediation. Adapted from Kavanaugh (1994).

ting the biodegradation rate constant (how fast bacteria degrade the pollutant) versus the hydraulic conductivity (the rate at which water can move through the aquifer materials). If the rate constant is very high, bioremediation is feasible. However, feasibility is also limited by hydraulic conductivity. Obviously, if the water will not move very fast, then neither the organisms nor the nutrients can move through the water, and effective bioremediation will not result. Hydraulic conductivity may be embraced with new technologies such as pneumatic fracturing, which attempts to break up aquifer materials and create paths for nutrients, organisms, and water to flow. The values given in Figure 9-3 are relative, and a more extensive database is needed so that we can better understand these limitations. Bioremediation works best in homogeneous aquifers and with compounds that are not overly hydrophobic. Hopefully, in the future, continued research will enable us to remove some of these limitations.

PROCESS FUNDAMENTALS

Microbiologists and others doing research in the biological sciences are well aware of what it takes to care, feed, and grow an organism, but engineers often need to be reminded. A general checklist of requirements for microbial activity is useful in this regard (Table 9-1). Additional details are given by Flathman et al. (1993), Gibson and Saylor (1992), Madson (1991), McCarty (1993), National Research Council (1993), Norris et al. (1993), Parkin and Calabria (1986), Thomas and Ward (1989), and Zitomer and Speece (1993). A few items are particularly important when trying to facilitate bioremediation. For example, items 1 and 2: organisms need a carbon and energy source to grow. This source may be found in the pol-

TABLE 9-1 Checklist of Requirements for Microbial Activity

---

1. Carbon source
2. Energy source (electron donor)
3. Terminal electron acceptor
4. Macronutrients (nitrogen and phosphorus)
5. Micronutrients (e.g., trace metals and sulfur)
6. Proper pH
7. Proper temperature
8. Absence or control of toxic materials
9. Adequate contact (bioavailability)
10. Adequate time
11. Desired microbes or genetic machinery

---

lutant to be removed. However, in some cases a growth substance needs to be added, which is an engineering challenge and an engineering cost. The terminal electron acceptor condition, or the nature of the environment, is very important. For example, if the growth of aerobic bacteria is desired, a source of oxygen must be provided.

Items 4 to 8 are environmental factors necessary for microbial growth. For example, many groundwaters are deficient in the macronutrients nitrogen and phosphorus. Many bioremediation schemes involve adding at least one of these nutrients. Items 9 and 10 are engineering variables. With in situ bioremediation, adequate contact, sometimes called bioavailability, is extremely important.

Essentially, we are trying to bring together three elements: the pollutants to be removed, the organisms, and the nutrients needed by those organisms. Without all three, bioremediation cannot be accomplished. It is a significant engineering challenge to promote adequate contact. Sufficient time is also required; usually time is not a big problem with in situ bioremediation because the retention time in aquifers is in the order of months or years, which is usually enough time to bring about these reactions. Finally, there is a need to have the desired microbe or genetic machinery to bring about the desired biological reaction. There is significant potential for future development here.

Compounds, especially xenobiotic compounds, can be biodegraded in two ways: as a primary substrate (electron donor or electron acceptor), where the organism is grown by degrading the organic compound, or by co-metabolism, where the organism does not obtain energy for growth from biotransformation of the organic compound. Co-metabolism is important for many xenobiotic compounds. Here, the organism does not get sufficient energy from the compound to grow, either because the concentration is too low or the organism cannot process the compound as a growth substrate. The compound may still be removed, but a primary growth substrate must be present. This, too, represents a significant engineering challenge.

Several types of microorganisms are used in bioremediation. The current applications of bioremediation generally make use of indigenous organisms (organisms already present in the groundwater environment). The growth of these organisms must be stimulated by adding nutrients, electron donors, and/or electron acceptors. Two other types of organisms that may be used are acclimated strains, which have been developed from naturally occurring organisms, and genetically engineered microorganisms, in which desirable traits from several strains of organisms are combined so that the organism becomes much more versatile. These organisms must survive and grow in situ to accomplish bioremediation. Therefore, one of our major tasks is to develop robust strains of organisms that will survive in the environments into which they are introduced. Use of genetically engineered microorganisms is probably years away, more likely for political rather than technical reasons.

SUCCESSFUL BIOREMEDIATION

To understand the current status of bioremediation, it is useful to list compounds that have been successfully bioremediated in laboratory-scale studies, pilot-scale studies, field-scale studies, and full-scale applications (Table 9-2). Most of our successes, both ex situ and in situ, have been with the first three categories of compounds: petroleum hydrocarbons; benzene, toluene, ethylbenzene, and xylene compounds (termed BTEX); and the other petroleum-type chemicals like alcohols. We are accumulating additional information and experience with the other chemicals listed.

Data in Table 9-3 and Figures 9-4 and 9-5 describe the current status of the use of bioremediation in the field. The first four technologies listed in Table 9-3 are considered to be established technologies, and it is no surprise that most remedial actions to date have used these technologies. The other listed technologies are considered to be innovative or emerging technologies. As of 1991, bioremediation was being used at approximately 9 percent of Superfund sites.

The Environmental Protection Agency (EPA) has developed a database called the Bioremediation Field Initiative (U.S. EPA, 1993), which is an attempt to catalog the use of bioremediation at not only Superfund sites, but also at other sites. The data in Figure 9-4 show that most bioremediation schemes are in the design phase.

Although bioremediation is most often applied to the petroleum hydrocarbons, chlorinated solvent wastes and pesticides are now also being bioremediated. The "other" category in Figure 9-5 includes compounds such as the nitroaromatics (e.g. trinitrotoluene, or TNT).

TABLE 9-2 Partial List of Compounds That Have Been Bioremediated

---

- Petroleum hydrocarbons (gasoline, diesel, jet fuel, oil)
- Benzene, toluene, ethylbenzene, and xylene (BTEX) compounds
- Alcohols, ketones, esters
- Polynuclear aromatic hydrocarbons (simpler ones such as naphthalene)
- Creosote
- Chlorinated aliphatic hydrocarbons
- CFCs
- Chlorinated benzenes
- Polycholorinated biphenyls
- Phenols and chlorinated phenols
- Nitroaromatics
- Pesticides (EDB, alachlor, atrazine, dinoseb)

TABLE 9-3 Superfund Remedial Actions (Through Fiscal Year 1991)

Technology	Number of Sites	Percent of Sites
Solidification/stabilization	128	26
Off-site incineration	85	17
On-site incineration	65	13
Other established	10	2
Soil vapor extraction	84	17
Thermal desorption	28	6
Ex situ bioremediation	25	5
In situ bioremediation	20	4
In situ flushing	16	3
Soil washing	16	3
Dechlorination	8	2
Solvent extraction	6	1
In situ vitrification	3	<1
Chemical	1	<1
Other innovative	3	<1
TOTAL	498	100

Source: Adapted from Kavanaugh (1994).

To understand and apply these processes more successfully in the future, we must demonstrate conclusively that bioremediation (i.e., biological processes) is responsible for the disappearance of these compounds. The National Research Council's Committee on In Situ Bioremediation (1993) offers three tests. First, there must be documented evidence that the contaminant is disappearing in the field. This task is relatively easy, with currently available samplers and analytical methods. Second, it must be shown that organisms at the site, or organisms to be introduced at the site, have demonstrated potential for contaminant biotransformation. One way to do this would be to take soil cores from the site, bring them to the lab, and in carefully controlled experiments demonstrate that bioremediation can occur. Third, and most difficult, is to provide conclusive evidence that bioremediation has actually occurred in the field. Several methods can be used: For example, organism concentration can be measured. If the organism concentration increases at the same time the contaminant decreases, then it is likely that the organisms are doing the biotransformation. The disappearance of the electron acceptor (e.g., oxygen) could be monitored. Oxygen disappearing when the pollutant disappears is circumstantial evidence that biotransformation is responsible for the removal. This type of information is particularly difficult to get in the field with present technology.

Bioremediation has been most successful with petroleum hydro-

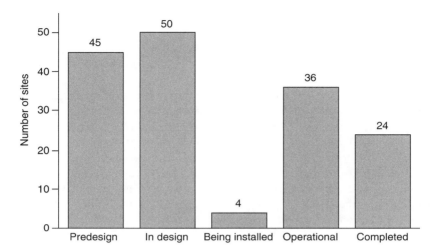

FIGURE 9-4 Bioremediation: status of operation. Adapted from U.S. EPA (1993).

carbons, even in Alaska at cold temperatures. The initial success was achieved by Richard Raymond in Pennsylvania, where there was a leak of 100,000 gallons of gasoline (Raymond et al., 1975). The free product was recovered by physical means and bioremediation was stimulated by adding ammonium sulfate, a phosphorus source, and oxygen via an air

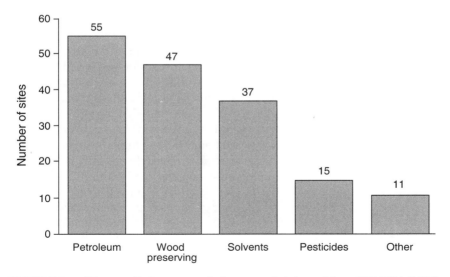

FIGURE 9-5 Bioremediation: wastes being treated. Adapted from U.S. EPA (1993).

sparger. Petroleum hydrocarbons were monitored and none were detected after 10 months. Data from core samples taken at the site showed that the concentration of organisms in the soil had increased at the same time the hydrocarbons had disappeared, proving that bioremediation occurred.

A second example is a California site where the soil and groundwater were contaminated with petroleum hydrocarbons (Norris and Dowd, 1993). Soil levels ranged from zero to 1900 ppm for total petroleum hydrocarbons (TPH) and up to 32 ppm for the sum of benzene, toluene, ethyl benzene, and xylene (BTEX) compounds. The groundwater levels for BTEX compounds ranged from near zero to more than 6,000 ppb; the drinking water standard for benzene, for example, is 5 ppb. The groundwater was remediated by using groundwater recirculation, the oxygen source added was hydrogen peroxide, ammonium chloride was added as a nitrogen source, and tripolyphosphate was added as a phosphorus source. Within 10 months the levels of TPH and BTEX in the groundwater and soil were below detection limits. Bioremediation was confirmed by noting that the disappearance of TPH and BTEX coincided with the disappearance of the added microbial nutrient, ammonia, and an increase in the carbon dioxide concentration of the soil gas and the groundwater. The presumption is that the increased carbon dioxide comes from the biodegredation of the petroleum hydrocarbons. Additional examples are given by Flathman et al. (1993), National Research Council (1993), and Norris et al. (1993).

To expand current understanding and applications of bioremediation, engineers need answers to several questions. They need to know what is being done, how it is being done, who is doing what, why is it being done, how fast it is being done, whether we can do it faster and better, whether we can control it, whether we can meet cleanup standards, and whether we can predict with reasonable certainty that what we want to happen will happen. It is very important that we be able to reliably predict success.

An example of a recent development answering some of these questions and taken to the field is the anaerobic biotransformation of perchlorethylene ($CCl_2=CCl_2$, PCE; also called tetrachlorethene). It has been known for at least 10 years that under anaerobic conditions PCE is reductively dehalogenated, first to trichlorethylene (TCE), then to dichlorethylene (DCE), then to vinyl chloride (a known human carcinogen), and finally, in some cases, to ethene. As each successive chlorine is removed, the reaction rate becomes slower. Thus, these less chlorinated compounds accumulate and appear to be very difficult to biodegrade further. However, aerobic organisms with oxygenase enzyme systems (e.g., methane monoxygenase and toluene dioxygenase) can co-metabolically degrade these less chlorinated compounds to carbon dioxide, chloride, and other products. These aerobic processes are quite expensive and have their own problems.

There may be hope for complete anaerobic treatment. Initial evidence was provided by research conducted at a Superfund site in St. Joseph's, Michigan, where there was a TCE plume (McCarty and Wilson, 1992). As the progress of the TCE plume was monitored, TCE decreased, DCE appeared and then began to decrease, vinyl chloride appeared and then began to decrease, and ethene was produced. Researchers at Cornell University investigating the degradation of PCE under anaerobic conditions with and without methane formation found that they could get PCE to degrade to ethene in the laboratory (Freedman and Gossett, 1989; DiStefano et al., 1992). In Europe researchers developed an enrichment from a contaminated river sediment that could dechlorinate PCE all the way to ethene and then to ethane (de Bruin et al., 1992). An organism was isolated from this sediment that uses PCE or TCE exclusively as an electron acceptor for growth (Holliger et al., 1993). This organism dechlorinates PCE and TCE to DCE, and then other organisms in the enrichment apparently convert DCE into ethane.

These exciting discoveries have been used in the field. At St. Joseph's, Michigan, because the conversion of TCE to ethene appears to be occurring more rapidly than the plume is leaving, the strategy is to allow natural bioremediation to occur in some TCE plumes. As a result of the work in the Netherlands, a full-scale above-ground facility (where hydrogen is added to facilitate the growth of the PCE-degrading organisms) is remediating PCE-contaminated waste. In a field-scale study conducted in Victoria, Texas, benzoic acid and sulfate were added to stimulate indigenous organisms that will convert PCE to ethene and ethane (Beeman et al., 1993). Side-by-side control sites demonstrated that bioremediation was responsible for the conversion that occurred. The plot that received benzoic acid and sulfate showed conversion of PCE into ethene and ethane, whereas the control plot that received no benzoic acid and no sulfate showed no PCE removal. Thus, recent developments in this technology are being quickly taken to the field.

LIMITATIONS AND FUTURE NEEDS

However, we must be careful not to move too quickly. Many limitations need to be overcome if we are to realize the full potential of bioremediation. It is perhaps useful to categorize the limitations and needs as engineering, basic and applied microbiology, and carefully controlled field studies.

Perhaps the most important engineering challenge is the need for better site characterization. We need inexpensive, efficient ways to determine the extent of aquifer contamination. We also need better methods of assessing, in the field, whether the potential exists for biotransformation of the compounds there. Techniques based on molecular biology (e.g., gene probes and immunoassays) may be very helpful here. If the contaminants are not bioavailable, they are not going to be bioremediated. We need to understand the effect of the nonaqueous-phase liquids (NAPLs) on the important microorganisms. How close can the organisms live to these liquids? We need better models both for screening and prediction. We need better scale-up methods, particularly in the field. How do we go from laboratory scale to pilot scale and then to field scale? How do we reasonably ensure success? Finally, there is a need for innovative process design: innovative reactor designs for ex situ systems and innovative delivery systems for in situ applications. There is much room for improvement here.

In basic and applied microbiology, there is potential for explosive improvement in bioremediation. Consider, for example, the discovery of new bacterial strains, such as the PER-K23 strain that uses PCE or TCE exclusively as an electron acceptor (Holliger et al., 1993). Such advances may be taken rapidly to the field, as described above. We need better understanding of microbial ecology and population dynamics in the environment and of how microbial ecology and these dynamics are affected by mixtures of contaminants. Rarely is a site contaminated with only one compound. With a better understanding of the pathways of degradation, perhaps we can control these pathways. We also need to better understand gene expression and manipulation in the field, and new tools need to be developed. For example, how does one tell whether genetic machinery is available at a site to bring about the desired reactions? There is significant potential here for probe techniques, for example, gene probes and immunoassays. There is potential for development of genetically engineered microorganisms and a general need for developing robust strains of organisms. Finally, there is even potential for bioremediation of some metals. For example, hexavalent chromium can be reduced to trivalent chromium, which is unstable and will precipitate as a solid, making it less mobile. It may be possible to reduce uranium(VI) to uranium(IV), which will precipitate as an oxide.

Finally, there is a need for more carefully controlled field studies. Such data would help address the problem of how to go from the laboratory to the field. The field studies at Stanford University offer a model (Hopkins et al., 1993; Roberts et al., 1990; Semprini et al., 1991). An interdisciplinary approach is needed that includes engineers, microbiologists, microbial ecologists, molecular biologists, hydrogeologists, chemists, etc. We need field studies that include side-by-side comparisons with controls. These field studies will help generate a more extensive inventory of bioremediation successes and failures. After all, successful engineering is basically the prudent use of these kinds of inventories. There has been some movement in this area. Two examples are the Advanced Applied Technology Demonstration Facility (funded by the Department of Defense) at Rice University and the field-testing initiative that is being coordinated by the University of Michigan at a site in Michigan.

With additional research and experience in the field, bioremediation will no doubt become an even more important treatment technology in the arsenal of technologies used to clean up our contamination problems. Bioremediation offers the promise of cost-effective, environmentally acceptable treatment of contaminated waters, soils, and sediments. There is much interest in and enthusiasm for this emerging biotechnology.

REFERENCES

Bakst, J. S., and K. Devine. 1993. Bioremediation: environmental regulations and resulting market opportunities. Pp. 11-48 in Bioremediation: Field Experience, F. E. Flathman, D. E. Jerger, and J. H. Exner, eds. Chelsea, Mich.: Lewis.

Beeman, R., S. Shoemaker, J. Howell, E. Salazar, and J. Buttram. 1993. A field evaluation of in situ microbial reductive dehalogenation by the biotransformation of chlorinated ethylenes. Proceedings of the 2nd International Symposium on In situ and On-Site Bioreclamation, San Diego, April 1993.

de Bruin, W. P., M. J. J. Kotterman, M. A. Posthumus, G. Schraa, and A. J. B. Zehnder. 1992. Complete biological reductive transformation of tetrachloroethylene to ethane. Appl. Environ. Microbiol. 58:1996-2000.

DiStefano, T. D., J. M. Gossett, and S. H. Zinder. 1992. Hydrogen as an electron donor for dechlorination of tetrachloroethylene by an anaerobic mixed culture. Appl. Environ. Microbiol. 58:3622-3629.

Flathman, F. E., D. E. Jerger, and J. H. Exner, eds. 1993. Bioremediation: Field Experience. Chelsea, Mich.: Lewis.

Freedman, D. L., and J. M. Gossett. 1989. Biological reductive dechlorination of tetrachloroethylene and trichloroethylene to ethylene under methanogenic conditions. Appl. Environ. Microbiol. 55:2144-2151.

Gibson, D. T., and G. S. Saylor. 1992. Scientific Foundations of Bioremediation: Current Status and Future Needs. Washington, D.C.: American Academy of Microbiology.

Holliger, C., G. Schraa, A J. M. Stams, and A. J. B. Zehnder. 1993. A highly purified enrichment culture couples the reductive dechlorination of tetrachloroethylene to growth. Appl. Environ. Microbiol. 59:2991-2997.

Hopkins, G. D., L. Semprini, and P. L. McCarty. 1993. Microcosm and in situ field studies of enhanced biotransformation of trichloroethylene by phenol-utilizing microorganisms. Appl. Environ. Microbiol. 59:2277-2285.

Kavanaugh, M. C. 1994. In situ remediation: research needs. Paper presented at AEEP Research Opportunities Conference, Ann Arbor, Michigan, September 20-22, 1994.

MacDonald, J. A., and B. E. Rittmann. 1993. Performance standards for in situ bioremediation. Environ. Sci. Technol. 27:1974-1979.

Madsen, E. L. 1991. Determining in situ bioremediation: facts and challenges. Environ. Sci. Technol. 25:1662-1673.

McCarty, P. L. 1994. In situ remediation. Paper presented at AEEP Research Oppostunities Conference, Ann Arbor, Michigan, September 20-22, 1994.

McCarty, P. L. 1993. In situ bioremediation of chlorinated solvents. Curr. Opin. Biotechnol. 4:323-330.

McCarty, P. L., and J. T. Wilson. 1992. Natural anaerobic treatment of a TCE plume, St. Joseph, Michigan, NPL site. Pp. 47-50 in Bioremediation of Hazardous Wastes, EPA/R-92/126. Cincinnati, Ohio: US EPA Center for Environmental Research Information.

National Research Council. 1993. In Situ Bioremediation. When Does It Work? Washington, D.C.: National Academy Press.

Norris, R. D., and K. D. Dowd. 1993. In situ bioremediation of petroleum hydrocarbon contaminated soil and groundwater in a low-permeability aquifer. Pp. 457-474 in Bioremediation: Field Experience, P. E. Flathman, D. E. Jerger, and J. H. Exner, eds. Chelsea, Mich.: Lewis.

Norris, R. D., et al. 1993. Handbook of Bioremediation. Chelsea, Mich.: Lewis.

Parkin, G. F., and C. R. Calabria. 1986. Principles of bioreclamation of contaminated ground water and leachates. Pp. 151-163 in Hazardous and Industrial Solid Waste Testing and Disposal, Sixth Volume, ASTM STP 833, D. Lorenzen, et al., eds. Philadelphia, Pa.: ASTM.

Raymond, R. L., V. W. Jamison, and J. O. Hudson. 1975. Biodegradation of high-octane gasoline in groundwater. Dev. Ind. Microbiol. 16.

Roberts, P. V., G. D. Hopkins, D. M. Mackay, and L. Semprini. 1990. A field evaluation of in-situ biodegradation of chlorinated ethenes: part 1, methodology and field site characterization. Ground Water 28:591-604.

Semprini, L., G. D. Hopkins, P. V. Roberts, and P. L. McCarty. 1991. In situ biotransformation of carbon tetrachloride, freon-113, freon-11, and 1,1,1-TCA under anoxic conditions. Pp. 41-58 in On-Site Bioreclammation, R. E. Hinchee and R. F. Olfenbuttel, eds. Boston: Butterworth-Heinemann.

Semprini, L., P. V. Roberts, G. D. Hopkins, and P. L. McCarty. 1990. A field evaluation of in-situ biodegradation of chlorinated ethenes: part 2, results of biostimulation and biotransformation experiments. Ground Water 28:715-727.

Thomas, J. M., and C. H. Ward. 1989. In situ biorestoration of organic contaminants in the subsurface. Environ. Sci. Technol. 23:760-766.

U.S. Environmental Protection Agency. 1993. Bioremediation in The Field. EPA/540/N-93/001, No. 8. Cincinnati, Ohio: US EPA Center for Environmental Research Information.

Wentz, C. A. 1989. Hazardous Waste Management. New York: McGraw-Hill.

Zitomer, D. H., and R. E. Speece. 1993. Sequential environments for enhanced biotransformation of aqueous contaminants. Environ. Sci. Technol. 27:226-244.

Part 3

FROM LABORATORY TO MARKETPLACE: THE CHALLENGES OF TECHNOLOGY TRANSFER

Technology transfer, the issue of how to translate scientific discoveries into useful, commercially viable products, is a focal point in the debate surrounding biotechnology. However, as Jerome Schultz, of the Center for Biotechnology and Bioengineering at the University of Pittsburgh, points out in Chapter 10, the issue is neither new nor unique to biotechnology.

In a historical review of relationships between universities (where most basic scientific research has traditionally been carried out) and industry (which tends to favor research oriented toward product development), Schultz notes that cooperation, as well as tension, between the two communities extends back to the earliest days of university involvement in research at the beginning of this century. Schultz argues that the explosion of government support for university-based research after World War II weakened university-industry collaborations because it became easier for academic scientists to apply for government grants than to build the relationships necessary to obtain funding from industry.

Both Schultz and National Science Foundation director Neal Lane, author of Chapter 11, argue that although there are indeed significant differences in the cultures of the academic and business communities, the extent of the gulf between the two groups has been exaggerated. Far from being ivory towers interested solely in the pursuit of knowledge for its own sake, Schultz and Lane say, universities have long recognized the need to connect "the discovery process" (as Lane calls it) with "the process of putting new discoveries to use."

Nevertheless, conflicts of interest are an inherent part of the research system, according to José Trías, vice president and general counsel of the Howard Hughes Medical Institute (HHMI) until his tragic death in May 1994. For example, where scientists value the free exchange of information because it promotes the advance of knowledge, business people see a need to protect product-related information to maintain an advantage over their competitors. In Chapter 12, Trías describes the approach taken by HHMI (the nation's largest private nonprofit supporter of biomedical research) to achieving a balance between the valid but often divergent interests of the academic and business communities.

Since 1980, when Congress passed the Bayh-Dole Act (P.L. 96-517) allowing universities to hold patents on discoveries made through government-sponsored research, the U.S. government has encouraged patenting to promote the commercial development of scientific discoveries. However, in Chapter 13, Rebecca Eisenberg of the University of Michigan argues that although patents may promote technology transfer in some circumstances, the adoption of a single approach to technology transfer fails to fully take into account the complexity and unpredictability of the scientific discovery process.

10

Interactions Between Universities and Industry

JEROME SCHULTZ

A recent survey of graduate deans revealed that one of the most critical issues facing their graduate programs is the question of university-industry interactions; these concerns are summarized in Table 10-1 (Morgan et al., 1993). There is a partial myth that a university is inherently an open institution, that all information generated at a university should be freely available to everybody. Because of this prevailing presumption, it is not unusual to hear comments to the effect that anything that sequesters information at a university is against the public's interest and therefore "bad."

Another perceived problem is that because of funding pressures, the research agenda of universities may be biased by industrial support to focus on "hot areas," which may be different from intellectually important problems. In the past 10 years, biotechnology, computers, and materials science have been some of the frontier areas in which industry has been supporting research. Sometimes ignored in these discussions is the pressure by other institutions, such as, groups in Congress, to prioritize the research portfolio of universities to meet perceived national needs. An example of this is Senator Mikulski's (1994) new emphasis on strategic funding: ". . . we should be spending more than half of our basic research dollars in areas we consider strategic. Our investments in science and science policy will become a new super highway of ideas and technology to achieve national goals."

Another area of concern is whether industry-related research efforts inevitably lead to the exploitation of students. The presumption is that

131

TABLE 10-1   Research Relationships Between Universities and Industry: Perceived Problems

For Universities	For Industry
• Intellectual property	• Minimal marketable products
• Conflict of interest	• Leakage of proprietary information
• Conflict of duties	• Excess monitoring required
• Consulting	• University research not timely
• Use of university facilities	• University not focused
• Secrecy	
• Focus on "hot" areas	
• Exploitation of students	

students working on projects that are generated by industry would be bound by contractual considerations, thus preventing them from pursuing their own creative research ideas. Does their educational experience suffer because of these factors?

Industry also has concerns. One is the perception that university faculty prefer to do curiosity-driven research that is often very far removed from marketable products. A related concern is that academic researchers drift from stated goals of their research programs to follow interesting leads with the hope of being first to uncover and publish on a new phenomenon.

Because much of university research is carried out by graduate students who have other obligations, such as course work, another problem is the difficulty that academic groups have in meeting project objectives in a timely fashion. Companies fear that their personnel may have to expend extraordinary efforts and time with their university colleagues to make sure that a joint project is moving along expeditiously.

Industry is also concerned with the leakage of proprietary information developed within the university's laboratories. It is in the company's interest to maintain certain information as proprietary, either for a patent application or for production purposes.

There are potential problems as seen from both sides in these interactions. For successful interactions it is absolutely necessary for both groups to be aware of these problems and to put procedures in place at the start of a project to prevent interferences in a productive relationship.

Many discussions of university-industry interactions tend to be colored by the patterns of a comparatively few "research" universities that dominate these scientific activities of the academic community. There are about 1500 colleges and universities in the United States. About 500 of them have graduate-level science departments but only about 200 are doctorate-granting institutions. Yet when one examines the size of the research faculty and the amount of research funding, about 100 schools qualify as research universities.

Research funding is concentrated in a relatively few universities. Eighty-five percent of the research funding—about $13 billion in 1992— goes to the 100 research universities, and 21 percent of that funding ($3 billion) goes to 10 universities. The focus here will be on these 10 universities; some of the research paradigms appropriate for these large institutions may not apply to others. Also, there are signs that even the 100 research universities may not be able to sustain their research activities over the next decade because of the need to replace and replenish existing facilities and equipment in the face of leaner federal budgets.

There is extensive diversity in research programs among universities. With the ever-present competition for all sources of funds—federal, state, industry, foundations—each institution seeks to establish its competitive advantage so as to distinguish itself from it colleagues and to be more attractive to supporting agencies.

DISTRIBUTION OF UNIVERSITY REVENUE

University-industry relations should be considered in the context of the budget of a typical university. For example, the University of Pittsburgh, a modest-size university, has many sources of funding (Figure 10-1). The size of these income streams indicates the potential effect of these factors on the pattern of university activities. It is not unusual that tuition and fees do not account for most funds needed to run a university. In this instance the research sector accounts for about 20 percent of the university's income, so although important, it is not the dominant factor in university revenue. Most discussions of university finances focus on tuition, state funds, and research grants as sources of revenue, but as can be seen for the University of Pittsburgh, roughly 30 percent of the money comes from other sources. Some universities are involved in auxiliary enterprises (e.g., real estate businesses and educational and other service facilities).

This brief overview illustrates that universities are business enterprises engaged in a variety of businesses. Although this discussion focuses on research, the importance of university-industry interactions should be considered as only one, most likely minor, component of the overall university budget. Averaged across all academia, present industrial support accounts for only about 8 percent of the total research expenditures at universities.

An additional component of university finances, not included in Figure 10-1, is the operation of the university medical center. Most research

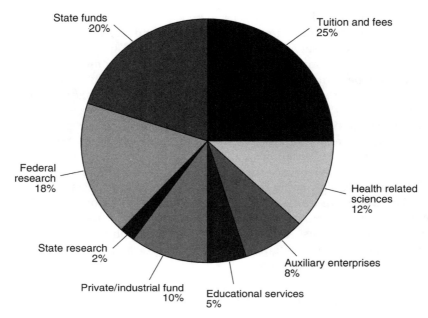

FIGURE 10-1 Typical distribution of university revenue.

universities have an associated hospital and medical center. The annual budget of these operations is usually the same size as that for the total academic enterprise and often is much larger. The health-related academic and service budget may be the dominant budgetary item in many universities and can have a tremendous effect on the nonhealth academic programs. Surprisingly, there is very little discussion in academic circles on the influence of the health-service enterprise on university planning and resources whereas industry-related issues are hotly debated.

A HISTORY OF UNIVERSITY RESEARCH

Initially, universities in the United States did not engage in any research. Universities were established basically for general education, i.e., language, religion, arts, and humanities; they were not established for research. As best as I can determine, university research in the United States started in the 1850s when land grant universities were established by Congress in response to society's need to develop technologies useful for agriculture and industry. This tradition of universities responding to society's needs continues today and must be appreciated to understand the evolution of the research agenda of universities.

Until the early 1900s the research activities of the land grant universities were slanted toward agriculture rather than industry. This neglect of industry-related research for about 50 years probably stemmed from the lack of funds from state governments to purchase and maintain the equipment necessary to set up industry-like manufacturing units. Universities could not afford the production or pilot plant facilities necessary for these types of efforts. The focus instead was on classroom teaching; the practical training of students was left to industrial employers to provide on the job. Hands-on experience that is required for a position with significant responsibility in the production aspects of industry is still not provided at school. Companies usually provide about 2 years of training in technology to an engineering graduate with a bachelor's degree in science. So although the intent of land grant legislation was to foster industry-university collaboration, the interactions with farmers prospered through the formation of university-based agricultural experiment stations.

The debate and conflict that consistently arises today in discussions on the meaning and value of basic vs. applied research goes back almost 100 years, and it is unlikely that any new cogent ideas are going to surface any time soon. The Massachusetts Institute of Technology (MIT) was one of the first universities to initiate research laboratories in the sciences in the early 1900s and also was the first university to experience the stress generated by divergent views on basic vs. applied research. In 1903 A. A. Noyes introduced the concept of providing research experience to broaden the training of students in university laboratories. He solicited and received foundation grants for the Research Laboratory of Physical Chemistry for conducting research within the chemistry department. W. Walker in the same department apparently considered the research carried out by Noyes as ivory tower research, not truly related to industrial needs. So he established another research laboratory—the Research Laboratory for Applied Chemistry—and obtained money from industry to study research problems. This might have been the first "job shop" in a university.

The conflict between Noyes and Walker was so strong that Noyes eventually left MIT and went to the California Institute of Technology, which marked the beginning of the chemistry department there. G. N. Lewis also left MIT's chemistry department and started the research activities at the University of California, Berkeley. The Research Laboratory of Physical Chemistry at MIT was disbanded in the 1930s and replaced by the Division of Industrial Cooperation, a subscription service that gave companies access to faculty resources. Disputes regarding the quality of research and loss of subscribers led to the guideline that sponsored research "must enhance the prestige of the institution, vitalize teaching, and provide helpful contacts for students."

MIT eventually handled this situation by sanctioning faculty consulting with industry, and this policy has been adopted by most universities. The presumption is that through consulting, faculty members learn about industrial needs and bring this appreciation of industrial practice to students through the university's education program.

NATIONAL RESEARCH COUNCIL

World War I was the next event that significantly affected the university research agenda. After the war, Vannervar Bush realized that universities were a resource for fundamental science, and the National Research Council was formed to coordinate federal needs with university research. This initiated the era of federally funded research, and since then the government has played the leading role in university research.

On the entry of the government into research funding at universities, a fundamental shift in the paradigm for the selection criteria for the recipients occurred. Whereas previously private foundations decided research support based more on the general reputation of the institutions and individuals, the National Research Council adopted the policy of supporting the best-qualified institutions and individuals. This seemingly innocent and reasonable modification of the selection process was the start of the peer-review concept in research funding, which has become an institution in its own right and has grown to be so cumbersome that today it unnecessarily consumes a major part of the energy and saps at the vitality of the research enterprise.

EFFECT OF WORLD WAR II

By the 1930s there were still only about a dozen research universities. World War II was the next national emergency that had a major effect on the research programs within universities. In response to the war effort and the increasing awareness of the importance of technology in that effort, universities were encouraged to form research associations to conduct government-sponsored military research (e.g., the Lincoln Labs at MIT and the Willow Run Labs at Michigan). The government-sponsored military-university complex succeeded because of the rapid infusion of funds during the war years. This contrasts with the previous century, when the attempted government promotion of university-industry activities (through land grants) was ineffective. During the war the federal government had a major influence on the university research agenda affecting physics (nuclear weapons), engineering (radar and communications), and microbiology (antibiotics). In many projects secrecy was essential, requiring drastic procedures, such as the isolation of research laboratories from the academic facilities. Universities accommodated themselves to the conduct of secret research, so that they now have over 50 years of experience in conducting research at various levels of security. Thus the recent concern that proprietary research is foreign to universities is largely unfounded.

After World War II, permanent federally sponsored research institutes at universities were established. For example in 1948 Stanford initiated the Steeples of Excellence program to obtain government (mostly classified) research support and developed government-funded microwave and electronics research laboratories. Excellent research capabilities at universities became attractive to industry, and some institutions seized on this new opportunity to further broaden their support from industry. Stanford was highly innovative by developing the concept of research parks situated near the university. Further, they initiated academic degree programs for part-time students to bring industrial researchers back into the university. Stanford also established some of the first industrial-affiliate programs and now has about 35 such programs.

There was another outgrowth of World War II and the perceived need to have a ready scientific capability for military purposes. Vannervar Bush, who was the head of the National Research Council under President Roosevelt, in 1952 helped to form the National Science Foundation (NSF) to support basic research. The infusion of funds into universities by the NSF focused the attention of the university science community on basic research and, indirectly, pulled academia away from industry collaborations.

THE SPUTNIK CRISIS

The initial funding of basic research at universities by NSF was modest, but with the launching of the Soviet satellite, Sputnik, in 1957, Congress became intensely concerned about the capability of the American research establishment. Increases in appropriations to federal agencies for the funding of research in universities rapidly escalated. One year after Sputnik, NSF's basic research appropriation was increased threefold to $137 million. These were the "easy money" times for universities. With this infusion of federal resources into research, the number of research universities rose from about 12 to the 100 we have today.

This expansion of federal funding further weakened university-industry relations. Obtaining industrial support requires a good deal of effort: companies with an interest in a specific research program have to be identified by the university's faculty. In turn these companies then have to be convinced that the potential outcome of the research project would be financially beneficial. For obtaining a federal grant, there are only a handful of funding agencies to approach and each agency directs the grant application to its most relevant program. A good deal of anonymity is involved and the faculty do not have to get involved with face-to-face marketing of their research ideas.

As the number of university positions expanded, graduates with doctorates preferred to go to a university rather than into industrial laboratories to pursue their professional careers. University positions are perceived to be more prestigious, and, additionally, faculty members are thought to have more freedom to pursue their own research agendas.

The growth in federal funding of universities continued unabated for more than 30 years until the present time. However, the justification for this funding has drifted from military preparedness to economic development.

CHANGE IN ECONOMIC THEORY

For the most part, the national concern with economic competitiveness and job creation appeared on the national agenda in the 1970s. During that decade a change in economic theory began to emerge. The major efforts of states to expand their job base traditionally had been directed to attracting divisions of mature companies, such as auto assembly plants. David Birch (1979), an economist at MIT, completed a study that suggested that small companies were the source of economic expansion. Birch studied more than 5 million firms to determine where jobs were created and how job creation could be stimulated. He found that most large companies shrank over the 10-year period of the study at the rate of about 8 to 10 percent a year. What this study showed was that if states wanted to produce more jobs, it would be wiser to look at small companies because 52 percent of the jobs came from small companies created within the previous 4 years. The small companies were, in this particular study, technology companies. Another study showed that small businesses commercialize innovations 24 times better than do large businesses, whatever the criteria, and that jobs grew nine times faster and output was three times larger than for large businesses (Osborne, 1988). The findings of this study, popularized by Pat Choate and Susan Walter (1983), eventually led to federal programs such as the Small Business Administration and the establishment of the Small Business Innovation Research grant programs.

Because of this change of paradigm to create more jobs, state governments and the federal government began to consider the promotion of innovation. Who is creating innovation and how could that innovation result in more jobs? To stimulate job creation through innovation, a number of states initiated financial support programs for technology development which naturally affected universities. Pennsylvania was one of the first with its Ben Franklin program; other programs followed quickly, such as the Edison program in Ohio and the CAT program in New York.

TABLE 10-2 Types of University-Industry
Cooperative Relationship

• Industry liaison-affiliate programs
• Consortia and special research centers
• Unrestricted and specific grants
• Contract and collaborative research
• Personnel (e.g., sabbatical) exchanges
• Consulting relationships
• University technology-transfer options
• Small-company counseling and support
• Joint ventures
• Research center funded by
  University and corporate supporters
  Federal government and industry
  State government and industry
  Industry trade associations

The basic premise behind these programs was to stimulate research and development in universities and promote cooperation with companies, particularity small companies, to help foster the transfer of technology to the industrial sector and thus to create jobs. This concept has become so pervasive that now there are more than 500 state technology programs. In the biotechnology discipline alone there are now 60 state biotechnology centers.

The three main technological areas targeted for job creation through innovation were biotechnology, computer technology, and materials science. Many states' programs stimulated businesses in those fields. Many new types of arrangements developed between universities and companies (Table 10-2). In the 1970s the industrial agenda and the university research agenda were forced together primarily by state initiatives to stimulate job creation. A recent survey showed that about 400 companies formed by MIT graduates employed 160,000 people and generated a gross income of $27 billion, which represents 20 percent of the state's gross income.

Birch's findings dominated public policy for the past two decades. Recent studies by Steven J. Davis (1994) of the University of Chicago indicated that the role of big business in job creation is equally important.

UNIVERSITIES ENTER THE TECHNOLOGY BUSINESS

December 18, 1980, was the watershed date that launched the current era of intense university involvement with industry. The Bayh-Dole Act (P.L. 96-517) allowed universities to have patent rights for government-sponsored research. The rationale behind this legislation was that billions of dollars of federal funds had been spent in sponsoring research at universities and few jobs had resulted, and legislators were looking for ways to put technology into practice. The federal government had been particularly ineffective at marketing intellectual property (patents) that came from their research support in universities. By giving universities commercial rights to their research innovations, it was expected that it would be in the best (financial) interests of the universities to promote technology transfer to industry. Thus more effective methodologies for commercialization and job creation would evolve.

Before 1980 the federal government spent about $30 billion per year on research and owned about 28,000 patents, but only 5 percent of these technologies were licensed. In that same era, universities obtained about 280 patents per year. By 1992 universities were obtaining patents at a rate of 1,600 per year and generating about $250 million per year in royalties. Data from the Association of University Technology Managers shows that markets of about $11 billion in product sales and 75,000 new jobs were created by the Bayh-Dole act.

Universities, however, were ill equipped to manage this new potential source of revenue. Universities began protecting their financial positions by encouraging faculty to file disclosures for patents. Because confidentiality and secrecy are essential in the early phases of the patenting process, there was a perceived violation of the "law" of free information access and communication within universities. In addition, stresses began to emerge between universities and industry because companies had been used to free access to faculty, students, and their research laboratories, particularly at publicly supported universities. Further, there was a perception (mistaken) that because most university research was supported by public money, any product of that research was in the public domain.

The emergence of this new role for universities prompted many debates, and one extreme position is exemplified by a statement of Derek Bok, president of Harvard University, who said the university's autonomy and integrity was threatened by "introducing to the very heart of the academic enterprise a new and powerful motive — the search for commercial utility and financial gain."

I do not think universities had changed at all. As noted earlier, universities have always been opportunistic and responsive to society. For example, in the 1980s NSF (under Eric Bloch's leadership) realized that its emphasis on pure science subsequent to the Sputnik crisis actually drove a wedge between universities and industry. NSF developed a number of programs to force a university-industry partnership. These programs, such as the engineering research centers and science and technology centers, require that the NSF-supported centers have an industrial component. These programs were based on NSF's previous successful experience with the university-industry cooperative research centers started in 1973. Universities readily subscribed to these initiatives. Hundreds of applications were processed by NSF, and well more than 100 grants were given.

Recent policy directives from university administrations and faculty indicate the extent to which university attitudes have accommodated to the societal and political dependence on universities as the engine of economic growth. In 1987 Pennsylvania State University faculty passed a resolution stating that some of the major roles of the university were to promote a business-sensitive environment, to promote economic development, and to encourage entrepreneurial activities. Today about 150 years after the initial foray of universities as institutions to promote economic growth, some universities, such as Boston University, are boldly acknowledging in public that business development is one of a university's roles in society.

RECENT "MEGA-AGREEMENTS"

Some examples of the extent of university participation in cooperative enterprises with companies are the number of "mega-agreements" initiated in the past 10 years (Table 10-3). These highly sought after (by universities) co-development business agreements were seen by some as the "golden calf" that would significantly support university research in the future.

Noticeably, most of these contracts were in the area of biotechnology. Why was that so? Possibly because of the coincidence that biotechnology was emerging as a technology about the same time universities were allowed to own property rights through the Bayh-Dole Act. Also, universities were the lead institutions in biotechnology research; thus, companies that wanted fast access to these technologies found a ready and willing partner in the university. Many faculty believed that these extensive and long-term agreements were the beginning of a new wave of research support for universities and would provide a stable source of funding without the continued harassment of peer review required by government-funding agencies. In fact, these mega-grants were awarded to only four institutions, so the pattern has not been widespread. Further, the mega-grant era is probably over. Some of these companies, such as Johnson & Johnson and Monsanto, have indicated that these arrangements did not work out for them as expected. They did not benefit as they thought they would, and it is unlikely that they will make such arrangements again.

NSF reports that industrial support of academic research and devel-

TABLE 10-3 Research and Development Agreements Between Academia and Industry

Institution	Company	Funds (In Millions)	Duration	Year Established	Area of Research
Mass. General Hospital[a]	Hoechst	$70.0	12 years	1981	Molecular biology
Scripps Research Institute	Johnson & Johnson	120.0	15 years	1981	Synthetic vaccine
Johns Hopkins U.	Johnson & Johnson	1.0	open	1982	Biology
Washington U.	Monsanto	100.0	12 years	1982	Biomedical research
Georgetown U.	Fidia Research Fdn.	62.0	open	1985	Neurosciences
Johns Hopkins U.	SmithKline Beckman	2.2	5 years	1988	Respiratory disease
Mass. General Hospital[a]	Shiseido	85.0	10 years	1989	Dermatology
Harvard Medical School	Hoffman-LaRoche	10.0	5 years	1989	Medicinal chemistry
Mass. General Hospital	Bristol-Meyers-Squibb	37.0	5 years	1990	Cardiovascular
U. of California at San Diego	Ciba-Geigy	20.0	6 years	1990	Arthritis
Scripps Research Institute	Sandoz	300.0	10 years	1992	Immunology, nervous system, cardiovascular disease

[a]Teaching Hospital Associated with Harvard U.

Source: Nicklin (1993).

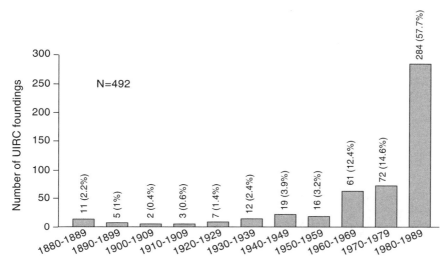

FIGURE 10-2   University-industry research centers (UIRC) founding, by decade, for centers active in 1990. Source: Cohen, Florida, and Goe (1991).

opment grew 50 percent, to $1.5 billion per year from 1989 to 1993. A recent survey of engineering research in U.S. universities showed that despite the disadvantages of industrial involvement with universities, 72 percent of the directors of organized research units in academia wanted more industrial involvement in their research programs (Morgan et al., 1993). Michael Crow at Columbia University said that about 35 percent of all patents issued to U.S. companies arise from collaborative research projects with universities (Hanson, 1994). The university-industry enterprise has reached significant proportions and must be considered a permanent component of university operations, at least for the research universities. Figure 10-2 shows the growth of university-industry research groups over the past 100 years.

The cost to universities of protecting their intellectual property is not insignificant. A 1990 survey of a dozen leading universities by Indiana University-Purdue University at Indianapolis showed the following average costs: intellectual property staff, one professional per $57 million in research support; average cost per staff member, $132,800 (not including patent costs); patent disclosures, four to five per $10 million of research grants and contracts; licensing and royalty income, 0.5 to 1.0 percent of total university research funding; and average income to university per license to industry, $18,000 to $28,000 (depending on maturity of the universities intellectual property office).

TABLE 10-4 Contrast of Research Cultures

University	Industry
• Research for knowledge and understanding	• Research to achieve competitive advantage
• Scientific achievement and public recognition	• Commercial significance and application
• Fast public communication	• Safeguarded proprietary information and delayed disclosure
• Free inquiry and flexibility to change directions	• Directed inquiry to company goals
• Cooperative and shared generic research	• Traditionally competitive
• New ideas, concepts, phenomena, and theories	• Applied research and technology development
• Leisurely pace with emphasis on thoroughness	• Urgent approach for business mission

CONTRAST OF RESEARCH CULTURES

Today we have a contrast of research cultures (Table 10-4). There is a perception that there are certain qualities expected of university research and others expected of industrial research and that these expectations are at two opposite poles. The two extreme views are that universities should pursue only pure, unrestricted research and that companies are only trying to get products to market. In fact, the attitudes of universities and businesses are actually coming closer together.

Roland Schmitt (1986), president of Rensselaer Polytechnic Institute, formerly at General Electric, and former member of the NSF board, perceives that the ideal relationship between the university and industry is a two-way flow of information. Schmitt believes it should be an arms-length relationship, where industry gives the university an understanding of the barriers that practice is facing but does not participate in the research. The university, in turn, provides the knowledge and talent needed to overcome the fundamental problems. The main goal is not to drive universities away from research, but to orient them toward the areas of fundamental research that are most needed by industry. There would be a definite separation of laboratories and personnel but an interaction by means of information transfer.

FUTURE DIRECTIONS

I think that universities and industry will be going in a new direction in the future, not the one proposed by Schmitt. There is a new economic paradigm, represented in part by Robert Reich's (1983) statement that "competitive advantage lies not in one-time breakthroughs, but in continual improvements." In industry the big breakthrough with the information explosion is not going to provide one company with an advantage over another company or one country with an advantage over another country. There will be a critical need for continuous interchange between the innovators and the producers. The innovators, who are at the university, somehow will have to be connected with the producers, who are in industry.

How might that happen? I think that universities will develop internal cooperative business-type organizations that interact with industry. Medical practice plans operating as businesses within the university are an example of this kind of organization. In industry a change in structure is resulting from the realization that passing technology from the research group to the production group does not work. Total quality management requires that the two groups be intimately interactive. The fundamental research groups in industry are disappearing, and industry is developing a need for what might be called "professional temporaries" in project-oriented teams.

John Armstrong, retired vice president at International Business Machines, stated that an essential component of effective technology transfer is the mobility of people (Hanson, 1994). Universities need to maintain a flexible research establishment so that industry can tap into the faculty as members of project teams. A faculty member would maintain a university appointment but would have a temporary involvement—a very close involvement—with business research. There are recent examples of the evolution of such research organizations at the University of Maryland and at Harvard University. The University of Maryland just opened a $53 million medical technology center in Baltimore that will house both academic and industrial scientists.

SUMMARY

Universities have responded to societal pressures and values. This adaptive nature of universities was nicely summarized by Susannah Hunnewell (1994) on the occasion of the announcement of the establishment of the Harvard Institutes of Medicine for developing innovative relationships with industry:

> Yet, in the light of the economic realities facing the university, perhaps Harvard's wrestle with its relationship to the private sector—the angel of good and evil—is simply a new stage in the evolution of academic values. A 1643 pamphlet stated that Harvard's mission was "to advance Learning and perpetuate it to Posterity, dreading to leave an illiterate

Ministry to the Churches." In 1708, amid much dissent, John Leverett became the first Harvard president who was not a clergyman, moving the University one step further from it theological mission and toward the secular academic code of ethics, which is now regarded as similarly unassailable. Perhaps technology transfer and implied partnership with industry—in Daniel Tosteson's words, "veritas brought to the sick and suffering"—will become a fundamental value of academia and of Harvard. However improbable it may seem now, such connections may even, someday, become inseparable from Harvard's mission as a disseminator of truth.

Universities do adapt to society's needs and they have changed over time. Universities do get involved in businesses and they can manage them very well. Universities and faculty have successfully managed proprietary research and they can do that very well. New organizational relationships with industry will be created. There are a number being tried and these kinds of relationships or organizational structures will be part of the university 20 years from now.

REFERENCES

Birch, D. 1979. The Job Generation Process. Cambridge, Mass.: MIT Program on Neighborhood and Regional Change.

Choate, P., and S. Walter. 1983. America in Ruins: The Decaying Infrastructure. Durham, N.C.: Duke Press Paperbacks.

Cohen, W. M, R. Florida, and W. R. Roe. 1994. University-Industry Research Centers in the United States. Pittsburgh: Carnegie Mellon University Press.

Davis, D. 1994. Quoted in myth: small business as job engine. Sylvia Nasor, NY Times, March 25, p. C I.

Hanson, D. J. 1994. Quoted in Budget realities usher in new era of research and development collaboration. Chem. Eng. News, Apr. 25, 1994., p. 35

Hunnewell, S. 1994. Harvard Magazine (Jan-Feb 1994), p. 3437.

Mikulski, B. 1994 In Forum on Science in the National Interest: World Leadership in Basic Science, Mathematics, and Engineering. Washington, D.C.: National Academy Press.

Morgan, M. E., D. E. Strickland, N. Kannankatty, and E. T. Rotto. 1993. Engineering research in U.S. higher education: characteristics, trends and policy options. Paper presented at the 27th meeting ASEE Midwest, Rolla, Mo., March 31, 1993.

Nicklin, J. L. 1993. University deals with drug companies raise concerns over autonomy, secrecy. Chronicle Higher Educ. March 24: A25.

Osborne, D. 1988. Laboratories of Democracy. Harvard Business School.

Reich, R. 1983. Pp. 324 in The Next American Frontier. New York: Penguin Books.

Schmitt, R. 1986. Pp. 19-27 in The New Engineering Research Centers: Purpose, Goals, and Expectations. Washington, D.C.: National Academy Press.

11

National Science Foundation's Perspective on University-Industry Interaction

NEAL LANE

In a rapidly changing field such as biotechnology, which touches the lives of people in so many ways, it is appropriate that we should devote a great deal of attention to the ethical concerns of industry-university relationships. All of us are aware of the increasing trend of establishing closer connections between the academic and industrial communities. The National Science Foundation (NSF) has served as a catalyst in developing models for how universities can do a better job of getting the best and the newest information out where it will do the most good.

There is a growing awareness that it is in the best interest of the research community to connect the discovery process, which is at the core of the academic world, to the process of putting new discoveries to use, which is the hallmark of successful industries. At NSF, we have encouraged this approach for quite some time with positive results. Nevertheless, developing partnerships between academe and industry, between discovery-driven research and market-driven technology development, is not without problems.

PARTNERSHIPS

One frequently noted source of problems is the different cultures of the two systems. The academic culture values openness and views itself as primarily driven by the pure desire for new knowledge, unswayed by prospects of personal financial gain (although a few academics have made some personal financial gain). The marketplace in its pure form has little

147

interest in investing significantly in knowledge for its own sake. Indeed, it has little room for other than economic concerns, such as maximizing profit, managing competition, and gaining market share, all understandable goals of business.

Both of these views fail to capture the remarkable complexity of the real world. Science and technology, universities and the private sector, have worked together for decades in mutually beneficial ways. Industry has a constant need for new information and for knowledgeable people familiar with the latest techniques. Academic researchers often find new scientific challenges arising from "real-world" problems, and it has been that way for a long time. More importantly, academia and industry have worked together in ways that have often strengthened the more positive aspects of the values of both: broadening the horizons of industry and focusing research on areas of practical consideration.

NSF-SPONSORED CENTERS

The possibility of mutually beneficial and noncompromising relations between academic researchers and industry is a basic assumption that underlies the success of more than 100 NSF-sponsored centers connecting universities and industry. Around the country, there are more than 1,000 centers and other collaborative organizations of this kind (Cohen et al., 1993). Research at the NSF centers ranges from telecommunications to steel making, from hazardous waste management to biotechnology.

So it is actually a myth that NSF has supported only the pure pursuit of knowledge, independent of any possible outcomes, and has shied away from encouraging its researchers to interact with industry and with states. It has a long-standing tradition of several decades of encouraging strong interaction with industry.

In the industry-university centers supported by NSF, both partners are beneficiaries of new information. Just as important, inasmuch as the primary responsibility of the university partner is education, the centers provide undergraduate and graduate students with a solid academic background plus hands-on experience with the practical problems of industry.

The umbrella provided by a center enables collaboration that might not otherwise occur. It creates an atmosphere where researchers can devote their energies to a small but important part of a larger problem related to their discipline or a joint project with another institution. These collaborations probably would not get started if they were left to a conversation at lunch or a corridor discussion at a scientific conference. They require much effort. They require champions on both sides. They require time and energy, both of which are precious, and a careful nurturing of the organizations involved in order to succeed.

It would have been comfortable for everyone never to have ventured beyond the university laboratories of independent investigators into the complicated world of collaborative centers. Many conflicts could have been avoided by serving only the interest of the academic researchers. However, more than 20 years ago, NSF took a chance on finding common ground between different cultures, and we have many successes to show for it. NSF provided the framework of incentives that enabled the different participants to come together. Despite the conflicts that do exist, these programs are having a profound effect on the culture of science and engineering. Multidisciplinary work is getting the attention it deserves, and many of the long-standing barriers between the industrial sector and the universities have begun to fall.

Most important, students are able to see the opportunities available in industry. There is another myth, at least in many disciplines of science, that universities actively discourage students from taking an interest in industry. It is suggested that what most professors do is attempt to replicate themselves so that they can be proud of their offspring, who will go out and do things similar to what they have done: teach and carry out research in major research universities around the country. Some data suggest that this does occur, but there are many examples of professors who have encouraged their students to work in a variety of careers.

SOME CHALLENGES

Universities could do more. We at universities and colleges could look harder at the educational opportunities we are providing. Are there situations in which we could help change student attitudes? Could we make clearer to students how their energies, abilities, and innovative skills could do more for society in jobs other than academic positions? Students are so sensitive to the views of their research advisors that it would not take much to show them that they would not be considered failures if they choose not to enter academia but to contribute to society in other ways.

Larger conflicts occur in these industry-university interactions, conflicts concerned with ownership of knowledge and equitable distribution of the benefits of academic research. These are difficult issues. The National Science Board's policy encourages maximum openness, reflecting the academic view that scientific information must be made widely available within the community. That ideal can run directly counter to the interest of industrial partners who may seek to protect new discoveries that their money has helped fund. NSF-sponsored centers have had success developing lasting intellectual property agreements between universities and industry and even between potentially competing industries working in the same center. It is not easy, but it can be and is being done.

Our experience has been that although intellectual property is a complex issue, it is an issue that usually can be addressed to the satisfaction of all partners. NSF has for the past two decades developed university-industry partnerships that have successfully dealt with the different values and objectives of the partners, addressed concerns about the ownership of intellectual property, and addressed potential conflicts of interest. Still, there are many possible pitfalls in future industry-university collaborations.

CONFLICT OF INTEREST

In the area of conflict of interest, NSF is in the process of publishing its policy on investigator conflicts of interest (NSF, 1994). The policy gives the primary responsibility for addressing potential financial conflicts of interest to the academic institutions, and NSF by and large would play no part. Institutions would establish their own policies, following these minimal requirements:

• The institutions would be required to collect financial disclosure information from investigators.
• The institutions would review the information to determine whether financial involvement might affect the objectivity of the researchers in conducting and reporting research findings.
• Institutions would take steps to minimize or eliminate any such risks and they would establish mechanisms for enforcing their policies.

In the areas of intellectual property and technology transfer, the basic NSF policy is federal law, namely the Bayh-Dole Act (P.L. 96-517 [35 U.S.C 18]). This law encourages the commercialization of new products developed with federal funds. NSF grantees are expected to seek patent protection and take steps to speed commercialization of inventions that result from NSF funding. If the awardee or the investigator does not wish to seek patent protection, NSF will make the opportunity available first to any other federal agency with an interest in the technology and then to the public.

The academic research community, as well as the industrial community, increasingly recognizes the benefits of carefully crafted collaborative efforts, but the university's primary mission is education, and that is challenging in itself. Whatever else the university does, it must not fail to educate well. We at NSF are confident that future partnerships between universities and industry, if they are based on mutual respect and careful consideration of each partner's responsibilities, can tremendously benefit both partners and the country as a whole.

REFERENCES

Cohen, W., R. Florida, and W.R. Goe. 1993. University-lndustry Research Centers in the United States: Final Report to the Ford Foundation. Pittsburgh: Carnegie Mellon University.

National Science Foundation. Fed. Regist. June 28, 1994.

12

Conflict of Interest in Basic Biomedical Research

JOSÉ E. TRÍAS

The great judge Learned Hand once said that justice is "the tolerable accommodation of the conflicting interests of society, and I don't believe there is any royal road to attain such accommodations concretely." What Judge Hand said of doing justice applies with equal force to protecting the integrity of basic biomedical research. Just as society must balance the rights of victims and the accused, of a free press and privacy, of free enterprise and public safety, and of free speech and national security, so we must balance competing interests in basic biomedical research. These conflicts are inherent to our research system. There is no practical way to avoid them nor is there only one way to resolve them. The best that universities and other research institutions can aspire to is, as Learned Hand said, "a tolerable accommodation." No royal road exists to attain those accommodations concretely.

Few challenges are greater than that posed by the complex and conflicting demands we place on our scientific enterprise. Consider, for example, the opening section of the Bayh-Dole Act of 1980. It calls for balancing our interest in promoting rapid utilization of inventions arising from federally funded research with our interest in promoting small business, U.S. manufacturing, collaborations between commercial concerns and nonprofit organizations, and free competition and free enterprise. Our interest in the integrity and vitality of academic research is not specifically mentioned but presumably is implicit throughout. We should also add competing institutional and individual interests to this competition of national interests. Singly, each interest represents a strongly held

152

value. Assembling them into a coherent whole makes for hard choices. None of us has a monopoly on wisdom or integrity in making these choices. We should regard the range of our approaches as a mark of healthy pluralism, not as a sign of weakness.

CORE PRINCIPLES OF RESEARCH

Those of us who conduct basic biomedical research in academic settings can agree on a few core principles. One is that the directions of basic research should be determined by sound scientific judgment, unencumbered by monetary concerns. Another is that the results of basic research should be published promptly and made available widely. Scientists who engage in basic research also should be free to talk with other scientists in both academic and industrial settings about new ideas, current or future research efforts, and other aspects of their work.

There also can be no argument about the importance of bringing the results of biomedical research expeditiously from the laboratory to clinical settings. When academic institutions and private industry work together to conduct biomedical research or to commercialize its results, the public stands to benefit not only through improved health, but also with new jobs and enhanced international economic competitiveness.

SUPPORT FOR RESEARCH

Industrial support for basic biomedical research can be invaluable in times of national budgetary retrenchment. Traditional sources of support for academic research these days are very tight. In recent years, the ratio of research project grant applications funded by the National Institutes of Health has been about one in four. In some institutes, fewer than one in five applications is supported. Funding from foundations and other nonprofit organizations is limited. Industrial support and collaboration, therefore, are essential to our biomedical research efforts.

Collaboration between industry and nonprofit organizations also has become a significant national objective, especially under the Clinton administration. The Bayh-Dole Act specifically authorizes use of the patent system to promote such collaborations, and federal income tax laws now clearly permit them.

Many prominent officials gathered in early 1994 at the National Academy of Sciences for a conference sponsored by the Office of Science and Technology Policy. Representative George Brown, who chaired the House Science, Space, and Technology Committee, said this at the meeting: "We cannot have a research system running on its own predetermined track and hope that it will intersect serendipitously with the needs of a dynamic, changing society. We must have, instead, a research system that arches, bends, and evolves with the society's goals." Senator Barbara Mikulski, who oversaw appropriations for several federal agencies that fund research, warned that "the U.S. is losing ground. The U.S. is losing time. And the U.S. is losing opportunities. To regain the ground we have lost over the last two decades, we must seek new models of collaboration between our universities and the private sector." Other speakers echoed the same theme.

The importance of academic-industrial collaboration also was made clear at the January 1944 meeting at the National Institutes of Health on conflict-of-interest issues inherent in the commercial sponsorship of academic research. In many ways this trend is welcome and overdue. Strengthening the ties between academic and industrial research will promote innovations of social value. Within the medical arena, the result could be needed funding of academic biomedical research and faster development of products that ease suffering and save lives. However, this trend also will accentuate and make it harder to balance this complex array of competing and conflicting national, institutional, and individual interests.

COMPETING AND CONFLICTING INTERESTS

Any restraint on the publication of research results impinges on academic freedom, and yet some restraint is required to protect patent rights and legitimate commercial incentives. Similarly, any commercial sponsorship agreement that lays out a particular research goal detracts from the principle that academic research directions should be determined solely by sound scientific judgment, but commercial sponsorship is an indispensable support for academic biomedical research. Moreover, an uncompromising insistence on protecting research directions from financial interest in every case would lead us to forbidding our faculties to hold stock in biotechnology companies, share royalties in licensed discoveries, and consult with industry. We are not prepared to do this.

Another conflict involves the public interest, so forcefully embraced by the Bayh-Dole Act, in having a research discovery brought to practical application by the company best able to do so. Because that determination is in most cases possible only after the discovery has been made, this interest is potentially threatened by any preexisting commitment that favors one company over another. Research arrangements between commercial sponsors and academic biomedical research labs almost always provide the sponsor with a preference over its competitors in commercializing discoveries that arise from the lab's research. The preference is often in the form of an option to license future discoveries, regardless of their commercial values, on terms negotiated before the discoveries were made. In some cases a very large fraction of the funding provided by the commercial sponsor is attributable to a preference of this kind. Where federally funded research is involved, this makes for a lively tension between two stated policies of the Bayh-Dole Act: to achieve the best practical application of a discovery and to promote academic-industrial partnerships. The resolution is not in sight.

One last conflict concerns restrictions on academic biomedical researchers discussing their work with others. Such restrictions may diminish academic freedom and retard scientific progress, but they also may be necessary to protect legitimate commercial interests in an academic-industrial collaboration. It is unclear whether the resolution of this conflict should rest with the individual scientists or with the collaborating institutions. Nothing short of a resolve by the government to free academic research from dependence on commercial sponsorship would avoid the conflict.

All of the conflicts just discussed, and not just this last one, are unavoidable given our institutional arrangements for funding and conducting basic biomedical research. We cannot practically change these arrangements or wish these conflicts away. We have to confront the conflicts and search for a balance that is appropriate for individuals, institutions, and the nation as a whole.

If Judge Hand is right, that means we must find tolerable accommodations. We must recognize that there is no easy, single way to arrive at these accommodations in every case, and we should welcome both a diversity of approaches and a disparity of accommodations. Perhaps our divergent solutions will never converge, but we should not fail, on that account, to exchange impressions.

HOWARD HUGHES MEDICAL INSTITUTE

In this vein, I would like to describe the role of the Howard Hughes Medical Institute (HHMI) in conducting basic biomedical research and the approach that it has taken in trying to balance these competing interests. HHMI is the nation's largest private nonprofit supporter of biomedical research by far, with an endowment nearing $8 billion. Last year it spent $268 million on biomedical research, an average of more than $1 million for each of its 225 investigators.

HHMI does not award research grants. It carries out basic biomedical research by employing its own scientists and their staffs and equipping their laboratories at more than 50 universities, teaching hospitals, and other academic settings (called host institutions) across the country. HHMI investigators concurrently hold faculty appointments at the host institutions. Like their faculty colleagues, in addition to conducting research they teach, mentor young scientists, and discharge other academic duties. For instance, Tom Caskey, Savio Woo, and seven other of our investigators have laboratories at Baylor University. There is an HHMI investigator at Rice, and there are 12 investigators in Dallas at the University of Texas Southwestern Medical Center.

HHMI investigators are appointed for terms of 3, 5, and 7 years, subject to reappointment after peer review of their work near the end of their terms. The attrition rate due to this process is less than one in five. This low attrition rate reflects the excellence of the scientists involved. HHMI's current 225 investigators include a number of Nobel laureates and more than 40 members of the National Academy of Sciences. Our philosophy is to support outstanding scientists for extended periods, not specific projects with limited time horizons.

We plan to add another 49 investigators, among them some of the nation's brightest young stars in biomedical research. We also employ and support research teams for each investigator. Altogether, there are nearly 2,000 people on our scientific staff. They do basic research focusing on cell biology, genetics, immunology, neuroscience, and structural biology. In addition, HHMI awards more than $50 million each year through its grants program, mainly for science education.

CONTRIBUTIONS OF HHMI INVESTIGATORS

HHMI investigators are making substantial contributions to elucidating fundamental processes that underlie health and disease. Ray White's participation in identifying the gene for an inherited form of colon cancer; Francis Collins's collaboration in the discovery of the gene for cystic fibrosis; Lou Kunkel's identification of the gene for muscular dystrophy; Bob Horvitz's participation in identifying a gene associated with familial amyotrophic lateral sclerosis, the inherited form of the disease that killed baseball star Lou Gehrig; Tom Caskey's participation in cloning an altered gene believed to be responsible for the most common form of inherited mental retardation, fragile X syndrome; Wayne Hendrickson's and Stephen Harrison's production, together with their colleagues, of the first three-dimensional image of the site on white blood cells (T cells) that acts as a target for human immunodeficiency virus, an image that could be helpful in designing drugs to prevent the virus from getting its critical foothold; and Mario Capecchi's development of gene targeting, a technique that has revolutionized genetic engineering and is now being used in laboratories across the country—all these and many other examples of extraordinary work—have been supported by HHMI.

This work does not go on in isolation from industry. HHMI encourages its investigators to form scientifically productive collaborations with private companies. We strongly encourage our investigators, through our host institutions, to commercialize the results of their research.

As of February 1944, HHMI investigators had recorded 469 discoveries with our office. Patent applications had been filed for 134 of these discoveries, and patents had been granted for 10 of them. HHMI also is involved in 65 licensing agreements. For example, one of our scientists at Yale, Richard Flavell, was among the leaders of a research team that made important discoveries about Lyme disease. Through a licensing agreement, SmithKline Beecham is now applying that research to develop a Lyme disease vaccine. Research by other HHMI investigators has led to diagnostic tests now used for sickle cell anemia and other genetic disorders. Mike Welsh, one of our investigators at the University of Iowa, is collaborating with a private firm on gene therapies for cystic fibrosis. David Williams, one of our investigators at Indiana University, is helping to develop therapies that will reduce the side effects of radiation treatment in cancer patients. HHMI investigators elsewhere are working with companies on research related to acquired immune deficiency syndrome, tuberculosis, and many other diseases.

This is a substantial record. It shows the importance that HHMI places on collaborating with industry and in transferring discoveries quickly from the research bench to the hospital bedside. In fact, our collaborations with industry extend well beyond licensing patented discoveries. Many HHMI investigators consult for private companies, hold stock in biotechnology ventures, or serve on scientific review boards of industrial concerns. A few investigators are founders of biotechnology concerns; most investigators regularly exchange ideas and biological materials with their counterparts in industry. HHMI investigators are engaged in scientifically important collaborations with biotechnology and pharmaceutical concerns. All of these interactions with industry are accommodated, usually successfully, by HHMI's policies on conflict of interest.

HHMI POLICIES ON CONFLICT OF INTEREST

HHMI investigators are expected to spend at least 75 percent of their time on research. The remaining time is available for teaching classes, serving on campus committees, and performing other academic duties. If professional time remains after discharging those duties, it can be used for consulting and for serving on scientific review boards of companies.

Investigators are required to sign a statement that assigns to HHMI all rights to any invention or discovery developed through research financed by HHMI. We work closely with our host institutions to commercialize these advances. If one of our researchers at Baylor makes a discovery, for example, we assign to Baylor all of the intellectual property rights. Baylor then takes the lead in seeking a patent and looking for licensees. We share with Baylor the costs of obtaining a patent. If there are royalties, we share those, too. The investigator's share is determined by the formula that Baylor uses for that purpose. The host institution takes the lead in commercializing the property, usually through a technology-transfer office, but HHMI monitors the process. We get copies of disclosure forms, initial patent applications, and so forth. We review license agreements with special care, because we want to be sure that the licensee's access to future research conducted in HHMI labs as a result of the license is limited to what is commercially reasonable to bring the specific discovery in question to practical application.

Collaborations between HHMI investigators and for-profit companies are welcome as long as they are driven primarily by scientific considerations. Our policy is that a company cannot simply pay for research that it hopes to commercialize. It must make a direct and substantial scientific contribution of its own, such as a process, a compound, or a laboratory technique. In short, HHMI's policies embrace scientific partnerships with industry but rule out commercially sponsored research arrangements.

Companies that enter into scientific collaboration agreements with HHMI reasonably expect some commercial benefit in return. When the situation warrants, HHMI will grant a company a time-limited option to license the fruits of the collaboration, but only on terms to be negotiated after the discovery is made. The firm also may receive a limited right of prepublication review to protect intellectual property, and its scientists may be allowed to work in an HHMI laboratory while supported by company funds. However, the company may not leverage the collaboration into broader rights to HHMI research.

We require our investigators to obtain written approval before entering into a collaboration with a for-profit company, even if the arrangement is proposed as a result of collegial and informal ties. Our experience is that the more informal the arrangement, the more likely it is that disputes will arise down the road, even if everyone starts off with the best of intentions.

We also require HHMI investigators to obtain prior approval for consulting agreements. Our researchers may not consult for a company in which they hold a significant equity interest. Generally this means 5 percent or more of the company's outstanding equity, but it depends on the circumstances. We sometimes consider a smaller percentage to be significant.

Consulting is limited to the exchange of ideas. An HHMI investigator may not conduct research for a company or direct others in doing so. Similarly, compensation for consulting may include fixed amounts of cash and equity but may not include incentive features, such as bonuses based on performance. We scrutinize high levels of compensation to ensure that payment is made only for the exchange of ideas and not to gain inappropriate access to HHMI research.

We consider the sharing of our biological materials to be an essential aspect of scientific citizenship. Our system enables our researchers to transfer materials to other academic and nonprofit laboratories with a minimum of paperwork. Transfers to for-profit labs require a bit more documentation but nothing burdensome. Our biggest concern in this area comes when one of our scientists accepts a transfer from a for-profit lab. Sometimes the agreements that accompany these transfers are too broad, claiming rights to almost anything that results. HHMI policies require that these agreements meet a test of reasonableness.

HHMI investigators are encouraged to seek outside funding from the government and from private philanthropic organizations. They may accept gifts from for-profit companies as long as they make no commitment to the sponsor in return.

Finally, HHMI investigators are required to conform to the policies of the host institution in addition to the HHMI policies just described. The result is to give dispositive effect in any case to the more restrictive policy. HHMI's policies resemble in many ways those of our host institutions. Indeed, our requirement that HHMI investigators conform to both HHMI and host institution policies works tolerably well precisely because, in many cases, the policy differences are not great. By delegating commercialization of HHMI discoveries largely to host institution policies and procedures, HHMI adopts, de facto, the principles and policies of the Bayh-Dole Act, thus indirectly embracing national interests such as the preference for small business, the U.S. manufacturing requirement, and the promotion of free competition and free enterprise. However, HHMI policies do differ from those of our host institutions in certain significant respects.

For example, as mentioned earlier, we have an explicit upper limit of permissible stock ownership in a company for which a HHMI investigator wishes to consult. We specifically disallow incentive compensation in consulting without exception. We restrict consulting to the exchange of ideas and flatly prohibit the conduct or direction of research for an industrial concern. In scientific collaborations with an industrial partner, we may agree to grant a preference to the industrial partner to commercialize the fruits of the collaboration, but we will limit the preference to an option to license on terms to be negotiated after the discovery is made. Some of our host institutions draw these lines in somewhat different ways. The sharpest difference is in our approach to commercial sponsorship of research. Academic research institutions, by and large, accommodate it. HHMI policy rules it out.

HHMI'S PHILOSOPHY

Our philosophy is to support outstanding scientists for extended periods, not specific projects with limited time horizons. We believe that the nature and extent of our support frees HHMI investigators to pursue basic biomedical research along directions determined by their own scientific judgment and to take unusual scientific risks. This freedom is expensive, but we believe it contributes to the vitality of our biomedical research enterprise and is worth the cost. We believe that the pressures inherent in commercial sponsorship could undermine this freedom. We rule out commercial sponsorship of HHMI research to protect this freedom.

Like our host institutions, however, we continue to evaluate and reevaluate our policies on conflict of interest. Academic-industrial interaction is increasing. The pattern of interaction is evolving. It would be sheer happenstance if policies fixed yesterday served us well tomorrow. Along with our host institutions, we believe that our labors in this area are not near an end.

13

Patents: Help or Hindrance to Technology Transfer?

REBECCA EISENBERG

"I ntellectual property" is a broad heading used to refer to a wide variety of rights associated with inventions, discoveries, writings, artistic works, product designs, and designations of the source of goods and services. Patents and trade secrets are the most important of these sorts of intellectual properties in the field of biotechnology.

One aspect of intellectual property that distinguishes it sharply from other forms of property—and for some people makes it harder to justify—is that intellectual properties may be possessed and used by many people simultaneously. This is not so for tangible property. If someone borrows my car, I cannot use it—nor can anyone else—until the car is returned to me, but if someone borrows my secret manufacturing process or my backup copy of my word processor, I can keep on using it while someone else is using it. In fact, no matter how many people I share my word processor with, as long as everybody can make a copy, it is not going to interfere with my ability to keep on using it. This capacity for simultaneous possession by many people is a feature that is common to all sorts of intellectual property, including computer programs, musical recordings, lists of customers, and self-replicating cell lines or genetically engineered organisms. Many people intuitively feel that they are doing nothing wrong when they make unauthorized use of intellectual property as, for example, when they borrow and copy other people's computer programs.

What, then, justifies a system of exclusive legal rights to ideas and

161

information that others could benefit from without depriving the owners of their use? In the United States, intellectual property is usually justified in instrumental terms, although some advocates of intellectual property try to justify it in moral or natural-rights terms. The instrumental justification for a patent system is that inventions and discoveries are often costly to make as an initial matter but cheap and easy to copy once someone else has made them. Because the public benefits from new inventions and discoveries, we want to encourage people to invest in research and development, but they might not be willing to do so unless they have some means of preventing competitors from reaping the benefits of their investment without sharing in the initial risk and cost.

SECRECY AS A WAY TO PROTECT INTELLECTUAL PROPERTY

One way of keeping inventions and discoveries out of the hands of competitors is to keep them secret. As long as no one else knows the company's formula, the company does not have to worry about competition from outsiders who did not share in the cost of developing it. However, secrecy only works for certain types of inventions, such as manufacturing processes, that can be exploited commercially without disclosure. Many inventions and discoveries are self-disclosing once you sell a product that incorporates them. Even if secrecy is feasible, it might not be desirable. We might want to promote disclosure of new inventions and discoveries in the interest of furthering continuing technological progress in the field.

PATENT PROTECTION

An alternative to secrecy for some inventions is patent protection. A patent gives an inventor the right to exclude others from making, using, and selling the invention for a limited term: 17 years from the date the patent is issued under current U.S. law, 20 years from the application filing date in many other countries. The inventor may choose to make, use, and sell the patented invention; license others to do so exclusively or nonexclusively; or suppress the use of the invention entirely. The one thing the inventor cannot do is to keep the invention secret. To obtain a patent it is necessary to file an application that includes a full disclosure of the invention and of how to make it and use it. In many parts of the world, this disclosure is made public 18 months after the application filing date. In the United States it is made public as soon as the patent is issued. Under either system, an inventor who wants to disclose the invention earlier can do so as soon as the patent application is on file without jeopardizing the prospects for getting a patent. So in addition to requiring disclosure, patents promote disclosure by providing a property alternative to trade secret rights that survives even after disclosure.

Advocates of patents believe that they promote technical progress both by providing economic incentives to make new inventions and to develop them into commercial products and by promoting disclosure of new inventions to the public. The extent to which the present patent system achieves these goals is not known. Few people would argue that invention and technical disclosure would come to a standstill in the absence of a patent system. Firms that introduce new technologies into the market might find some research and development profitable even without patent rights. The lead-time advantage over competitors gained by being first in the market with an innovation, for example, might be enough to justify continued expenditures on research and development.

COSTS OF THE PATENT SYSTEM

The prospect of obtaining patent rights undoubtedly increases incentives to invest in research and development, at least in some fields, but the social costs associated with having a patent system have to be weighed against these benefits. The most obvious social cost associated with patents is that they create monopolies that increase the price and reduce the supply of products that are covered by patents. This may be a tolerable cost for socially useful inventions that would not have been made without the incentives of the patent system—we might choose to have these inventions at a high price rather than not to have them at all, but it is a high price to pay for inventions that would have been developed even without patent rights.

It is therefore important to formulate rules of patent law that exclude from protection inventions that would have been made even without the added incentive of the patent system. Most patent systems attempt to do this by requiring that an invention have a certain level of importance before it can be patented. In the United States we require that an invention be new, useful, and nonobvious to be patented. The nonobviousness requirement is a mechanism for distinguishing between inventions that would come about without the patent system and those that need its added incentive. These rules are very difficult to administer and result in a lot of uncertainty in the patent system.

Patent systems also entail considerable administrative costs. These include the costs of determining which inventions are patentable, an activity that consumes the time and energy of technically trained people who might otherwise be adding to the knowledge base more directly. Patent applications also incur costs in procuring and enforcing patents, and their competitors incur costs in avoiding infringement (including the costs of research efforts aimed at inventing around patented inventions).

Patents may also inhibit inventive activity of people other than the patent holders in fields that are dominated by patents. Patents may distort social priorities by diverting resources toward invention and away from other social problems. They may distort research in favor of making patentable inventions and away from areas in which patent protection is not available, such as basic research or discoveries in fields that are excluded from patent protection but might nonetheless be socially beneficial.

THE PATENT SYSTEM IN BIOTECHNOLOGY

These costs of the patent system should be remembered when considering the role of patents in biotechnology, particularly the role of patents in publicly funded biotechnology such as the Human Genome Project (Eisenberg 1994a,b). The Human Genome Project is an interesting example because it involves extensive government funding directed toward generating vast amounts of information in the hope that that information will ultimately be put to use in developing new products and processes for the diagnosis and treatment of human disease. Much of this information is generated in government and university laboratories that are not in a position to undertake the research and development necessary further downstream to translate basic research discoveries into commercial products.

PATENTING AS A WAY TO PROMOTE
TECHNOLOGY TRANSFER

Technology transfer to the private sector is a prerequisite for the development of genome-related products, but how to achieve technology transfer in such a project is a complex matter. U.S. policy since 1980 has reflected an increasingly confident presumption that patenting discoveries made in government-sponsored research is the most effective way to promote technology transfer and commercial development of those discoveries in the private sector. Policy makers of prior generations may have thought that the best way to achieve widespread use of the results of government-sponsored research was to make them freely available to the public. Advocates of the new patenting strategy stress the need for exclusive rights as an incentive for industry to undertake the further costly investment necessary to bring new products to market.

This new strategy is justified in terms of both trade policy and technology policy. The trade policy argument is that although the United

States leads the world in basic research and the creation of new technologies, other nations do a better job of commercializing and adopting new technologies in the private sector. As a result, U.S. firms lose sales to foreign manufacturers of goods that are based on technologies pioneered in the United States. The competitiveness of U.S. firms in world markets might be enhanced by leveraging U.S. strengths in research into a stronger position of dominance in applied technology.

The technology policy argument is that government-sponsored basic research discoveries that have been left in the public domain have not been picked up by the private sector and developed into commercial products, or at least not at the rate that one would hope to see. If the economy needs a steady infusion of new technologies to grow and to improve worker productivity, many argue that we need to induce the private sector to tap into the wealth of new information emerging from government and university research. This rationale presumes that inventions made freely available are languishing in government and university archives rather than being actively exploited by all.

NEW PATENT POLICY OF THE 1980s

The solution to these twin concerns, in keeping with the privatization ethos of the 1980s, was to offer up the results of government-sponsored research for private appropriation by U.S. industry through the mechanism of licenses under government- and university-owned patents. Exclusive patent licenses from a government agency or university would make it profitable for U.S. industry to develop products that would be too risky or costly to pursue if the discoveries were left in the public domain and competitors were therefore free to enter the market once it was established. Technology transfer facilitated by patent rights would generate new products for U.S. consumers and create jobs for U.S. workers while protecting U.S. firms from foreign competition.

Curiously, although the primary motive behind this patent policy appears to have been a desire to benefit U.S. industry, the primary impetus to get it enacted into law seems to have come from the government, with the support of universities, rather than from the private sector. Although industry has been slow to go for the bait of patent licenses to government-sponsored research discoveries, the government has not wavered from the patenting strategy but has instead fortified it by extending it to cover more discoveries made in a wider range of research settings.

Starting in 1980 the presumption in favor of patenting research discoveries was applied to small business and nonprofit organizations making research discoveries with federal funding under the Bayh-Dole Act. In 1983 these provisions were extended by a Presidential memorandum to large businesses doing government-sponsored research. They were extended by statutory amendments to discoveries made at government-owned, contractor-operated facilities in 1984, then to intramural research and research performed under agreements between government agencies and the private sector under the Federal Technology Transfer Act of 1986. Subsequent legislation and executive orders have continued to broaden and fortify this policy.

Today we have a system that virtually guarantees that wherever federally sponsored inventions are made—whether in government, university, or private laboratories—anyone involved in the research project who wants the discovery to be patented may prevail over the objection of anyone who thinks the discovery should be placed in the public domain. Thus, for example, if a university is reluctant to patent a discovery made in its laboratories with federal funds, the sponsoring agency may insist on obtaining a patent. If a government agency or university has no interest in pursuing a patent, the investigator who made the discovery may step in and claim patent rights. If anyone sees money to be made through patenting a government-sponsored research discovery and has the resources and sophistication to pursue patent rights, chances are it will be patented.

QUESTIONING FEDERAL PATENT POLICY

Now all of this makes sense if we want all government-sponsored research discoveries to be patented. But do we? Since 1980 federal patent policy has assumed that discoveries left in the public domain will not be used and that granting exclusive rights to discoveries to businesses will ensure their commercial exploitation for the benefit of consumers, taxpayers, and the economy. Our present statutes come close to reflecting a conclusive presumption that this is so. But is it so in fact?

The answer probably will vary from one field to the next and from one discovery to the next. The strong pro-patent tilt of current policy seems like a vast oversimplification of the enormously complex task of achieving technology transfer across the broad spectrum of discoveries emanating from federally sponsored research.

One reason for the complexity is that technology transfer requires extensive back-and-forth communication among different types of institutions and among researchers and technology users who speak to each other across significant cultural divides. The extent of this problem varies among fields. In some fields, researchers in government and university labs share norms of openness that conflict with commercial interests in secrecy. Patent rights may sometimes reduce this difficulty by providing intellectual property rights that survive disclosure. At other times, concerns about preserving the ability to patent future discoveries might fortify commercial incentives to maintain secrecy and thereby aggravate the conflict between the cultures of academic research science and industry. Any policy that promotes widespread patenting of the results of government-sponsored research would thus need to take into account and manage the effect of patents on the research enterprise.

Even setting aside the culture of academic research and focusing exclusively on the perspective of industry, current policy seems to oversimplify a complex problem. Patents may make sense as a means of facilitating technology transfer for some government-sponsored discoveries, but there are reasons to suspect that they make little sense for others. The course of scientific discovery and product development is infinitely complex, variable, and unpredictable. Uniformity in technology transfer policy may therefore be a false ideal. Neither the old-fashioned approach of leaving all new discoveries in the public domain nor the newer approach of assigning exclusive rights in such discoveries to private parties should be uniformly applied across the entire range of publicly supported discoveries. In our eagerness to avoid the inadequacies of the public domain approach, we may have moved too quickly and too emphatically in the opposite direction to the point where patent rights in some government-sponsored discoveries may actually be undermining rather than supporting incentives to develop new products and bring them to market.

NIH APPLICATIONS FOR cDNA PATENTS

One sign of trouble in paradise for federal technology transfer policy was the reaction of industry trade groups a few years ago to the filing of patent applications by the National Institutes of Health (NIH) on thousands of partial cDNA sequences of unknown function identified in government laboratories (Eisenberg, 1992). The research that led to the controversial patent applications consisted of taking randomly selected cDNAs from a human brain tissue cDNA library and finding the DNA sequence for small portions of those genes without knowing what proteins or functions are associated with the genes. Beginning in the summer of 1991, NIH filed patent applications claiming the partial cDNA sequences as well as the full genes of which they are a part, which NIH claimed could be readily obtained with the partial sequence information. An avowed purpose of seeking these patent rights was to be able to offer licenses to firms to promote the development of products related to the sequences.

Some of these patent applications were rejected by the U.S. Patent and Trademark Office, and the new leadership of NIH decided not to appeal the rejections and to withdraw the remaining claims. Although the immediate controversy was thereby resolved, it is nonetheless worthwhile to reflect upon this controversy as a case study of the role of patents in technology transfer. These patent applications generated considerable controversy among scientists throughout the world who charged that the human genome represents the universal heritage of humanity and should be dedicated to the public domain. They argued that intellectual property rights could undermine scientific collaborations and thereby retard progress in the Human Genome Project. Much of the controversy within the scientific community has been a reprise of an old debate about the effect of intellectual property rights on research science norms.

What was striking about this controversy was that the patent applications were also opposed by trade groups from the industry that NIH intended to benefit through technology transfer. These trade groups are not composed of naive, idealistic scientists who have limited experience with patents and limited interest in product development. Their members are the same hard-nosed, profit-maximizing firms that the government is trying to entice into developing products out of government-sponsored inventions. Position statements from the Pharmaceutical Manufacturers Association and from two biotechnology trade groups that have since merged, the Industrial Biotechnology Association and the Association of Biotechnology Companies, expressed views on the NIH patent applications that contradict the hypothesis that patent protection for those particular discoveries was necessary to protect the interests of firms that might develop related products in the future.

The Pharmaceutical Manufacturers Association and the Industrial Biotechnology Association urged that NIH not seek patent protection on DNA sequences with unknown biological function but instead place such sequences in the public domain. The third group, the Association of Biotechnology Companies, supported the NIH decision to seek patent protection, but only as a means of generating revenues for the government and not as a means of ensuring the availability of exclusive rights to those sequences. Indeed, even the Association of Biotechnology Companies urged that the patents be licensed on a nonexclusive basis so as not to block development projects in industry. So although this position is nominally consistent with current federal patent policy, it contradicts its underlying rationale by conceding that, at least in this particular case, exclusive rights to the discoveries could interfere with their effective commercial development.

INDUSTRY OPPOSITION TO NIH PATENTING cDNA

Why might U.S. industry object to NIH's pursuit of these patent rights and what does that tell us about the role of patents in technology transfer? First, an easy explanation is that the firms may not want NIH to be in a position to grant or deny licenses to develop genome-related products. There is an essential irony in using government-owned patents to achieve technology transfer. This strategy places a government agency in a licensing role for the purpose of promoting privatization. If NIH holds patent rights to a significant portion of the human genome, it may use its position as licensor to regulate the development of genome-related products, which is the last thing that industry wants.

Exclusive licenses under NIH patents until recently included reasonable-pricing clauses that permit NIH to monitor the reasonableness of prices charged for licensed products. Exclusive and nonexclusive NIH licenses include domestic manufacturing clauses requiring the licensee to manufacture products in the United States or at least granting a preference for U.S. manufacture. Such provisions tie the hands of industry and limit the profitability of products developed even under an exclusive patent license.

Firms may be particularly wary of NIH as a licensor in view of its recent role in authorizing a generic drug manufacturer to pursue NIH's claim against Burroughs Wellcome to patent rights in the use of the drug azidothymidine (AZT) in the treatment of acquired immune deficiency syndrome. This episode highlights the ambivalence of NIH toward profit maximization in the marketing of health-related products.

Second, the patent rights that NIH sought may have seemed unnecessary as a means of protecting the profit expectations of industry. The current government patent policy is based on a simple model of technology transfer in which a patent on a government-sponsored invention is the only source of exclusivity on the horizon for firms seeking to develop related commercial products. However, commercial products in industries that make use of patents, such as the pharmaceutical industry, typically embody multiple patented inventions. If a firm has its own patent rights in a product that are adequate to protect its market position, NIH patent rights covering the same product or covering inventions that are necessary to develop or market the product may be nothing more than an annoyance to the firm. If government patents are not only unnecessary to provide market exclusivity, but also come with burdensome restrictions on pricing and place of manufacture, firms may see them more as a regulatory hurdle than as an incentive to innovation.

Third, NIH patents may have seemed ineffective in protecting the market position of innovating firms. Patent rights are most likely to be effective in promoting product development when they ensure the patent holder of a commercially effective monopoly in the relevant product market. Whether NIH patents would have had this effect depends on the scope of patent rights NIH had been able to obtain from the Patent and Trademark Office. Generally, the most effective commercial protection, and therefore the most powerful incentive to invest in product development, is provided by a patent on an end product that is sold to consumers. Partial cDNA sequences of unknown function may turn out to be marketable as end products—perhaps in a diagnostic product—but it is more likely that they will be useful as research tools to find the full-length genes to which they correspond and to make the products for which those genes code.

The NIH patent applications included claims to these full-length genes on the theory that, by disclosing how to use the partial sequences as probes to find the full genes, NIH had provided an enabling disclosure of how to make those full genes. Although the NIH patent application did not disclose either the complete DNA sequence for the genes or the proteins for which they code, it did provide a general description of how to use the partial sequences as probes to find the full genes and how to achieve expression of the gene products once the full genes have been found. But under recent court decisions it is unlikely that NIH would have been able to obtain patents on the full genes without setting forth their full sequences (see, e.g., *Fiers v. Sugano*, 984 F.2d 1164 [Fed. Cir., 1993]). Thus, NIH patent rights would probably have been limited to narrower claims to the specific partial cDNA sequences than are actually set forth in the applications. Such limited patent rights would probably not have been broad enough to give effective commercial protection to firms seeking to bring related products to market, and the argument for obtaining patents as a means of promoting product development would lose its force.

PATENTS ON RESEARCH TOOLS

The partial cDNA sequences themselves are primarily useful as tools for research and development. Not only is it difficult to detect and prove infringements of such patents, but often the only effective remedy even for proven infringement will be damages, because an injunction against future use of the invention at that stage would not thwart the efforts of a competitor who has already finished using the invention. One could argue for a substantial damage remedy, but as long as the competitor no longer needs to use the patented invention in the manufacturing stage, an injunction against future infringement would not serve to keep the competitor off the market. Firms that are interested in developing end products for sale to consumers are unlikely to see patents on research tools used only during research and development as an effective means of promoting their market exclusivity in the ultimate products. Such patents may generate royalty income for their owners, and the prospect of earning royalties may make it more profitable to develop further research tools in the private sector. However, it is unlikely to enhance the incentives of firms to develop end products through the use of those research tools.

I think there are reasons to be wary of patents on research tools apart from their ineffectiveness in promoting product development. Negotiating licenses for access to research tools may present particularly difficult problems for would-be licensees who might not want to disclose the directions of their research in its early stages by requesting a license. Moreover, a significant research project might require access to many research tools. If each of these tools required a separate license and royalty payment, the costs and administrative burden could mount quickly.

Patent holders, moreover, may find it more lucrative to license research-tool patents on an exclusive rather than nonexclusive basis and in the process choke off other firms' research and development. For years this country has sustained a flourishing biomedical research enterprise in which investigators have drawn heavily on discoveries that their predecessors left in the public domain. Even if exclusive rights enhance private incentives to develop further research tools, they could do considerable damage to the research enterprise by inhibiting the effective use of existing tools. Patents on research tools may offer ineffective commercial protection to firms that use the tools to develop new products for consumers while interfering with research and development within those firms.

The more research that remains to be done to develop a product, the more likely it is that the innovating firm will make further patentable inventions of its own. These subsequent inventions are more likely to be incorporated in the final product, and patents on such inventions are thus likely to be far more important to the firm's profit expectations than exclusive access to any particular research tool.

CONCLUSION

The present policy of promoting patents on federally sponsored inventions has become rapidly entrenched in U.S. law, although it is not clear that this policy always serves its underlying agenda of furthering the transfer of new technologies to the private sector for commercial development. Patents undoubtedly have a critical role to play in facilitating technology transfer in some contexts, but they can also interfere with technology transfer and with the broader goal of promoting continuing technological process. These goals may sometimes be served by allocating new information to the public domain. Government is uniquely situated to enrich the public domain, and we should be wary of disabling the government from performing this critical function in our eagerness to enhance private incentives to put existing discoveries to use.

REFERENCES

Eisenberg, R. 1992. Genes, patents, and product development. Science 257:903-908.

Eisenberg, R. 1994a. A technology policy perspective on the NIH gene patent controversy. University of Pittsburgh Law Review 55:633-652.

Eisenberg, R. 1994b. Technology transfer and the genome project: problems with patenting research tools. Risk: Health Safety Environ. 5:163-175.

Part 4

EITHICS, BEHAVIOR, AND VALUES
IN SCIENCE AND SOCIETY

E thics, behavior, and values are difficult, sensitive issues about which sincere, well-meaning people may disagree violently. Are there absolute standards of right and wrong that cannot be compromised under any circumstances, or do right and wrong represent the endpoints of a continuum, with most human actions falling somewhere between the two extremes? According to what standards does a pluralistic society judge new technologies that offer many potential benefits but also raise many ethical questions?

In this section authors with a variety of perspectives tackle a range of thorny ethical issues relevant to biotechnology: the values that individual scientists bring to their work, the way that work is judged by regulatory agencies and by the public, the way society responds (or should respond) to scientific discoveries, and the effect of value judgments within science itself.

Most scientists struggle to articulate their professional values, notes ethicist Judith Swazey of the Acadia Institute, yet young scientists are expected to implicitly absorb these values through associating with advisers and mentors. Swazey argues that this "osmosis strategy" is no longer enough and that scientists have a responsibility to train their students in the ethical conduct of research.

The nature of scientific misconduct and the way scientists are disciplined for alleged misconduct is examined by lawyer Barbara Mishkin of Hogan & Hartson, who contends that existing processes for dealing with allegations of scientific misconduct generally leave much to be desired and that a uniform federal policy is sorely needed to define scientific misconduct and establish general principles for investigating and sanctioning scientists.

In Chapters 16 and 17, the focus shifts from the behavior of scientists to the response of society to scientific discoveries. Scientist Daniel Koshland, Jr., of *Science* magazine and ethicist Mark Rothstein of the Health Law and Policy Institute at the University of Houston offer contrasting views of the implications of biotechnology for the general public. Koshland challenges conventional wisdom about many of the questions raised by biotechnology. He calls for an informed debate between scientists and the general public about the applications of biotechnology, arguing that in a pluralistic society no individual or group can set moral standards for everyone.

Rothstein zeroes in on the implications of genetics technology, including invasion of privacy, unequal access to services such as prenatal genetic testing, and the specter of eugenics. Where Koshland sees the impact of biotechnology on society as mostly positive, Rothstein sees it as a mixed bag that may create as many problems as it solves. He is clear, however, that the fundamental issue is not the existence of the technology but rather the values that society brings to bear on decisions about how the technology is used.

Finally, Ruth Bulger of the Henry M. Jackson Foundation for the Advancement of Military Medicine offers a wide-ranging critique of the values implicit in the way science has traditionally been conducted. The cumulative effect of these assumptions, she says, has been to exclude women from most clinical research trials. These notions must be re-examined, Bulger contends, to ensure that women as well as men benefit from advances in technology.

14

Ensuring the Ethical Conduct of Research: Who Is Responsible?

JUDITH P. SWAZEY

One of the ethical challenges that science and engineering face today, and doubtless will face in the twenty-first century, is ensuring that research standards and practices are of the highest possible ethical caliber. The question posed in the title is rhetorical: everyone involved in the research enterprise is involved.

I want to discuss two interrelated topics. First, why do I and others believe that we need to address the ethical conduct of research far more seriously and vigorously than has been done by most individuals, institutions, and professional organizations? Second, what means could be used to meet this responsibility? For the sake of simplicity, the term science as used here refers to science and engineering and their many subdisciplines, recognizing that there are many differences as well as similarities in their cultures and conventions.

PROFESSIONAL VALUES

The Acadia Institute is studying the education and socialization of graduate students, particularly the professional values they are acquiring and the ethical issues they are encountering during their training. Our databases include nationwide surveys of 2,000 faculty and 2,000 doctoral students in chemistry, civil engineering, microbiology, and sociology departments at major research universities, and in-depth interviews in eight departments. Various sets of our findings support the premise that if we are serious about the integrity of science, we need to pay closer attention to the nature of the professional values that undergird the work of researchers, to the types of ethical problems that researchers and their trainees are encountering, and to how those problems are (or are not) being addressed.

As we found in our interviews, scientists have trouble articulating their professional values or norms. Although those values embody their assumptions about the way research should be conducted, they usually live out those values without thinking or talking about them and transmit them implicitly rather than explicitly to the trainees who are their scientific heirs. The traditional norms of science were explicated in a classic paper by sociologist Robert K. Merton (1942). Merton described four norms that form the prescriptive basis for assumptions about appropriate research behavior across disciplines and institutions: 1) universalism: the separation of scientific knowledge from the personal characteristics of scientists, 2) communality: the sharing of research techniques and findings with all other scientists, 3) disinterestedness: the separation of research from personal motives for the sake of truth and the advancement of knowledge, and 4) organized skepticism: the critical, public examination of scientific work. These norms, in Burton Clark's (1983) words, "comprise not only the ethos of modern science . . . but also much of the ethos of the academic profession." This ethos, as Rosenzweig (1985) observes, "is something in the nature of a cultural myth. . . . Like all myths that are central to a culture, it has a firm basis in reality, but it exaggerates reality in order to serve its real purpose, which is to tell people how they ought to behave, not how they do behave."

Even prescriptive norms are seldom held by all members of a group, and actual behavior is even less likely to always be in conformity. More importantly, there is evidence that significant changes have been occurring in the normative structure or ethos of science, reflecting changes in working relationships among scientists, research foci and funding, etc. In a study of Apollo moon scientists, for example, Mitroff (1974) observed that the culture of their work was based on a set of norms point for point so opposite to the Mertonian norms that he termed them "counternorms:" particularism, solitariness, self-interestedness, and organized dogmatism.

In the Acadia study, we asked faculty and students about the extent to which they believe that each of the Mertonian norms or the counternorms should represent the behavior of scientists and the extent to which they believe they represent the actual behavior of faculty in their department. Overall, graduate students strongly support the traditional Mertonian norms as statements of how scientists should behave. However, substantial numbers of students subscribe to the counternorms, with some significant differences by discipline, gender, and citizenship between adherents to the two sets of norms (Anderson and Louis, 1994).

Few faculty strongly support the counternorms as replacements for the traditional norms, but only 20 to 25 percent strongly support the traditional norms of universalism, communality, and organized skepticism and only 5 percent strongly support disinterestedness. The clearest pattern emerging from our analysis of faculty subscription to the norms and counternorms is that a very high percentage of faculty are ambivalent: 50 percent or more for each of the value pairs (norm and counternorm). Their responses indicate that they believe that there should be a more complex neotraditional value system that incorporates the counternorms (Louis et al., in press).

If we believe that the ethos of science is an important shaping force for the conduct of research, it is important for those in the scientific enterprise to engage in some values clarification. They need to understand the norms they are subscribing to and think about whether those norms constitute the values framework they want to serve as a guide for their work. Otherwise, as Mark Twain said, "we don't know where we're going, but we're on our way."

ETHICAL PROBLEMS IN RESEARCH

One of our project publications reporting survey data on the perceived extent of ethical problems in graduate departments of programs received considerable attention in professional publications and in the media in this country and abroad and a voluminous amount of letters, phone calls, and faxes (Swazey et al., 1993). Our analysis grouped ethical problems into the three categories used by the Panel on Scientific Responsibility and the Conduct of Research (1992): scientific misconduct, questionable research practices, and other misconduct. According to the faculty and doctoral students responding to our surveys, cases of what they perceive as scientific and other forms of misconduct and questionable research practices are not rampant in academic research. However, our findings—which I must emphasize are not incidence figures—indicate that these problems are more widespread than many people have assumed. Science certainly is not riddled with research misconduct, consisting of the now well-known trinity of falsification, fabrication, and plagiarism, but neither are these misbehaviors extremely rare. For example, 8 percent of faculty and 7 percent of student respondents reported that they have observed or have other direct knowledge of plagiarism by faculty in their own department, and nearly 33 percent of the faculty have first-hand knowledge of student plagiarism. Instances of data fabrication by faculty were reported by 6 percent of faculty and 9 percent of student respondents.

Compared with their encounters with what they judged to be scientific misconduct, both groups reported knowing about more instances of what they perceived as ethically questionable research practices. For example, 22 percent of faculty knew of departmental members who have overlooked the sloppy use of data, 33 percent knew of cases of inappropriate assignment of authorship credits, and more than 40 percent knew of colleagues who inappropriately used university resources for personal purposes. Substantial numbers of encounters with other types of misconduct also were reported, such as ignoring policies for research with animal and human subjects and biosafety, sexual harassment and discrimination, and cheating by graduate students in course work.

Our study confirms the widely held view that fear of retaliation for reporting suspected wrongdoing is a key problem in the way that ethical problems are dealt with in universities. More than 50 percent of the graduate students would expect retaliation if they reported suspected misconduct by a faculty member, and 29 percent also would expect sanctions for reporting another student. Faculty also are concerned about the consequences of whistle blowing: only 60 percent believe they could report a graduate student and 35 percent believe that they could report a colleague with impunity. Faculty and students interviewed gave personal examples of why they are hesitant to confront or report someone they believe is engaging in ethically wrong or dubious research practices. Some said that even if they had compelling evidence of what they viewed as serious misconduct, they would not do anything because it was not their responsibility.

As has been recognized for many years, we need to change the social and ethical climate of academia and other work settings that makes it so perilous to engage in good-faith reporting of suspected wrongdoing. It is equally the case, as Barbara Mishkin (1994) argues forcefully, that we need to deal with the problems of misguided or bad-faith charges of misconduct being filed and then being egregiously mishandled by institutional committees and administrators.

One of the most cherished cultural values of academics and other professionals is the right to exercise collegial self-regulation or governance. In keeping with this strongly held value, 99 percent of the faculty who responded to our survey believe that academics should exercise collective responsibility for the professional conduct of their students, and 94 percent believe that they should do so for their colleagues. However, there is a vast chasm between what faculty members believe they should do and what they say they and their colleagues actually do. Only 27 percent of faculty members judge that their departments actually exercise a great deal of collective responsibility for their students' conduct, and only 13 percent believe that they and their departmental colleagues exercise substantial responsibility for each other's professional behavior. Thus, our findings indicate that in practice, personal autonomy takes strong precedence over a norm of collegial governance among academic researchers, as it does among other professional groups, such as physicians.

More than 80 percent of the faculty and students we surveyed believe that learning how to deal with ethical uncertainties, pressures, and problems, such as conflicts of interest, intellectual property rights, authorship and publication issues, and misconduct, should be an important component of graduate education. Yet, only a very small number (4 percent of faculty and 3 percent of students) think their departments actually take a very active role in such training. A major reason for this huge divergence between "should" and "does" is the faculty's strong belief that the most effective ways for students to learn about the professional values and ethical standards and issues in their fields are by interacting with faculty in research work and by informally discussing ethical problems when they arise during that work. This is the traditional way in which graduate students have been expected to assimilate knowledge of ethical standards and practices in their fields: by an osmosis-like diffusion from master to apprentice. However, this tradition rests on an assumption that is challenged by our study and other work: that every doctoral student has a mentor, or at least an active advisor, who attentively and carefully guides the student's work and plays an important part in professional socialization. Students whom we interviewed wished they had a mentor or a research advisor who spent more time with them in the lab or was available and willing to discuss their concerns about pressures to "churn out data" with little regard to its quality and how to deal with problems ranging from whether they should be a coauthor on a paper to gender and ethnic discrimination to cheating. It is a fallacy to equate an advisor with a true mentor or even to assume that advisors are truly advising their students. We also cannot assume that the osmosis strategy is sufficient for providing students with a sound grasp of the increasingly complex ethical issues involved in research, let alone a thorough grounding in the standards and practices of responsible research.

THE NEED FOR EDUCATION ABOUT RESEARCH ETHICS

This thesis opens onto another topic: the need for explicit, planned, and structured education about research ethics, an enterprise in which both faculty and students should think of themselves in the double role of teachers and learners, mutually engaged in analyzing, discussing, and attempting to deal with complex issues that often have no ready solution. Even scientific misconduct is not a simple matter about which there is little to be said except that it is wrong. As Weil (1993) stresses, "teaching has to include some attention to the elements of misconduct" because defining what constitutes falsification, fabrication, and plagiarism and determining whether they have occurred often "turns out to be less straightforward than one might expect."

There are many obstacles to teaching research ethics, not the least of which are arguments by skeptical scientists that such teaching is "unnecessary, unhelpful or even counterproductive" (Lo, 1993). Another barrier is the understandable apprehension that many science faculty feel about venturing into the unfamiliar terrain of applied ethics. We need more faculty training seminars to equip scientists to learn the content and methods of teaching research ethics. Faculty and administrators also must find ways to incorporate explicit attention to research ethics into their departments, such as required curriculum or laboratory time that go beyond the occasional lunch discussion or talk by an imported ethicist.

Our findings raise serious issues about the ethical environments in which teaching and research are conducted and about the content of the professional values and ethical standards that are being transmitted to graduate students. Our study is by no means the only work that points to the reasons for and importance of explicit attention to ethical issues in science and engineering. These matters have been addressed for years by many individuals and by professional societies such as Sigma Xi, which published its pioneering "little red book," *Honor in Science*, in 1984. During the 1980s, several highly publicized cases of scientific misconduct catalyzed developments such as the 1989 requirement of the National Institutes of Health that trainees supported by National Service Research Award institutional grants must receive instruction in the responsible conduct of research and stimulated several important studies and publications by the National Academy of Sciences complex (Institute of Medicine, 1989; National Academy of Sciences, 1989; Panel on Scientific Responsibility and the Conduct of Research, 1992).

On February 4, 1994, the Councils of the National Academies of Science and Engineering and the Institute of Medicine issued a concerned statement on scientific conduct (Councils of the National Academy of Sciences, 1994). They emphasized the responsibility of all participants in the scientific enterprise (individual researchers, universities and other research institutions, professional organizations, and government) to "continue to work with vigor to reduce the occurrence of practices that undermine the integrity of the scientific process" and call on all the participants "to renew [their] commitment to strengthening the professional climate of the research system." The councils affirm that "research mentors, laboratory directors, department heads, and senior faculty are responsible for explaining, and requiring adherence to, high standards."

As part of the social contract that exists between scientists and American society, scientists have been granted many privileges, including public financial support for their work and a large degree of autonomy in setting ethical standards and in governing the conduct of their professional groups. As researchers and teachers, in turn, they have a responsibility to ensure that they do not use that autonomy to ignore ethically wrong or questionable practices by colleagues or students or shirk their responsibility to train their students in the responsible conduct of research.

ACKNOWLEDGMENT

This project is cosponsored by the American Association for the Advancement of Science Committee on Scientific Freedom and Responsibility, the Council of Graduate Schools, and Sigma Xi and supported by grants 8913159 and 9222889 from the National Science Foundation. The following National Science Foundation components provided funding to the Ethics and Values Studies Program for support of the project: the Directorate for Social, Behavioral, and Economic Sciences, the Directorate for Biological Sciences, the Directorate for Engineering, the Directorate for Mathematical and Physical Sciences, and the Office of the Inspector General. Any opinions, findings, conclusions, or recommendations are those of the author and do not necessarily reflect the views of the National Science Foundation.

REFERENCES

Anderson, M. S., and K. S. Louis. 1994. The graduate student experience and subscription to the norms of science. Res. Higher Educ. 35:273-299.

Clark, B. R. 1983. The Higher Education System: Academic Organization in Cross-National Perspective. Berkeley: University of California.

Councils of the National Academy of Sciences, National Academy of Engineering, and Institute of Medicine. Statement on scientific conduct, Washington, D.C., Feb. 2, 1994.

Institute of Medicine. 1989. The Responsible Conduct of Research in the Health Sciences. Washington, D.C.: National Academy Press.

Lo, B. 1993. Skepticism about teaching ethics. Pp. 151-156 in Ethics, Values, and the Promise of Science. Sigma Xi Forum Proceedings, February 25-26, 1993. Research Triangle Park, N.C.: Sigma Xi.

Louis, K. S., M. S. Anderson, and L. Rosenberg. In press. Academic misconduct and values: the roles of productivity, entrepreneurship and department climate. Rev. Higher Educ.

Merton, R. K. 1942. Science and technology in a democratic order. J. Leg. Polit. Sociol. 1:115-126.

Mishkin, B. 1994. The needless agony and expense of conflict among scientists. Chronicle Higher Educ. Feb. 23:B1-2.

Mitroff, I. 1974. Norms and counter-norms in a select group of the Apollo moon scientists: a case study of the ambivalence of scientists. Am. Sociol. Rev. 39: 579-595.

National Academy of Sciences. 1989. On Being a Scientist. Washington, D.C.: National Academy Press.

Panel on Scientific Responsibility and the Conduct of Research; National Academy of Sciences, National Academy of Engineering, and Institute of Medicine. 1992. Responsible Science: Ensuring the Integrity of the Research Process. Vols. 1 and 2. Washington, D.C.: National Academy Press.

Rosenzweig, R. M. 1985. Research as intellectual property: influences within the university. Sci. Technol. Hum. Values 10:41-48.

Sigma Xi. 1984. Honor in Science. Research Triangle Park, N.C.: Sigma Xi.

Swazey, J. P., M. S. Anderson, and K. S. Louis. 1993. Ethical problems in academic research. Am. Sci. 81:542-553.

Weil, V. 1993. Teaching ethics in science. Pp. 243-248 in Ethics, Values, and the Promise of Science. Sigma Xi Forum Proceedings, February 25-26, 1993. Research Triangle Park, N.C.: Sigma Xi.

15

Misconduct: Regulating and Investigating Scientific Research

BARBARA MISHKIN

Law is the codification of our combined conventional wisdom after we achieved a reasonable concensus on basic principles. I am going to discuss general principles in the area of scientific misconduct that we have all agreed to or should have agreed to. I shall also review some of the issues that are viewed as scientific misconduct that I think are actually disputes among scientists and require guidelines.

It has been 20 years since the National Commission for the Protection of Human Subjects of Biomedical and Behavioral Research was established. Some issues looked at and then set aside as being premature for full consideration are resurfacing today, such as research involving human embryos, genetic screening, and genetic interventions.

THE POPOVIC CASE

Serendipity played a large role in the career of one of the scientists I recently represented, Mikulas Popovic. He was one of the people who studied the avian sarcoma virus, an animal retrovirus, in Czechoslovakia a number of years ago. Serendipitously, he came to Bob Gallo's lab at the National Cancer Institute when few other people believed that retroviruses could infect humans, and he happened to be there at the time when acquired immune deficiency syndrome (AIDS) became an urgent public health problem. Dr. Popovic was one of the people centrally responsible for making the blood test for human immunodeficiency virus (HIV) possible. That is when serendipity ended for Mikulas Popovic. He was caught in a scientific misconduct investigation that, contrary to all the rules and regulations, became very public, and that followed procedures incompatible with due process. During 4 years of investigations by various offices within the Department of Health and Human Services (HHS), Dr. Popovic had no opportunity to confront or cross-examine witnesses. He had no opportunity even to know what they had said. He had no opportunity to examine documents that were being used against him.

Finally, the HHS Departmental Appeals Board (DAB) heard his case and we had 12 days of what was, essentially, a trial. We were finally able to respond to the accusations against Dr. Popovic and to challenge the witnesses and the evidence relied upon by the HHS Office of Research Integrity (ORI). The panel of the DAB thoroughly vindicated Dr. Popovic (HHS, 1993). ORI believes that this opinion has turned everything upside down, changed the definition of scientific misconduct, required ORI to meet a higher burden of proof than it would have to meet otherwise, and caused endless problems in their handling of subsequent cases.

That is not my view at all. The DAB merely made ORI adhere to the definition of scientific misconduct that has been in the HHS regulations since 1989, and made it meet its burden of proof. When ORI was required to do that, it could not prove its case.

ORI has since announced that it intends to try to change what it believes the DAB did to its ability to prove cases (e.g., Anderson, 1994; Bivens, 1993; Charrow, 1994). ORI says it will propose new regulations to deal with the question of intent, for example, in the definition of scientific misconduct. If ORI cannot change the situation by amending the regulations, it plans to accomplish change through legislation. ORI would tell Congress that without its help, the office cannot operate.

DEFINITIONS OF SCIENTIFIC MISCONDUCT

HHS regulations define scientific misconduct that is of concern to the federal government as fabrication, falsification, plagiarism, and a fourth category, which includes activities that "seriously deviate from accepted practices in proposing, conducting, or reporting scientific research" (42 C.F. R. § 50.102.). The definition includes another sentence, which ORI neglected: "Scientific misconduct does not include honest error or honest differences in interpretation of data." ORI argued that any false statement, or any statement that was in error, in and of itself constituted scientific misconduct. That allows for no "honest error," but we all make mistakes. (Even ORI made mistakes, in their various pleadings and documents before the DAB.) Nevertheless, ORI insisted that any kind of error in a published scientific paper constitutes scientific misconduct. The DAB ruled that ORI's view is inconsistent with the regulatory definition of scientific misconduct, which expressly does not include honest error (Re. Mikulas Popovic, 1993).

The DAB also noted that ORI's interpretation was inconsistent with the current definition of scientific misconduct at the National Institutes of Health (NIH). Mikulas Popovic was in the intramural research program at NIH when he performed the research in question. Although NIH did not have a published definition of scientific misconduct in 1983 and 1984, they did publish intramural research guidelines in 1990 that refer to scientific misconduct as "fabrication, falsification, plagiarism, or other practices motivated by intent to deceive" (NIH, 1990). This is the closest that we could come to any definition of scientific misconduct, generally accepted within Dr. Popovic's scientific community, that applied to the intramural research program at the NIH during the 1980s.

The DAB ruled that ORI could not prevail in its accusations against Dr. Popovic unless it could prove that any errors in his paper were of such significance that they would amount to scientific misconduct as judged by scientists in his own community (NIH) in 1983 and 1984. Witnesses at the hearing testified that in 1983 and 1984, no scientist would have believed that anything other than intentional falsification, fabrication, or plagiarism constituted scientific misconduct. Because there were no regulations or guidelines in place defining it otherwise, that was the definition the DAB applied in reviewing Dr. Popovic's work.

BURDEN OF PROOF

The DAB requires that scientific misconduct be proven by a preponderance of the evidence, meaning that the amount of evidence supporting a finding of misconduct must be greater than the contrary evidence. To prove the case, ORI had to have 50.1 percent of the evidence on its side, as against 49.9 percent of the evidence that we could adduce. This is the least rigorous standard in the law, and ORI did not have the evidence to meet it.

In the end, the definition of scientific misconduct (although hotly contested over the 12-day hearing) was not determinative because the DAB concluded that ORI did not prove, by a preponderance of the evidence, that the disputed statements or data were even untrue, much less that there was intent to deceive. Thus, the DAB stated that even if they agreed with ORI (which they did not) that unintentional errors in insignificant details in a paper would constitute scientific misconduct under the 1989 definition, they would not have reached a different result (Re. Mikulas Popovic, 1993).

ORI later claimed that the DAB had ruled that any errors in the paper also must have a certain materiality or significance. The DAB did not make any such ruling. They examined the errors that ORI asserted were in that paper and noted that even ORI's own witnesses said they did not affect the findings of the reported research. They did not diminish at all the robustness of the findings or the persuasive array of data that were published.

So the question became: What motive would anyone have to falsify data that are so insignificant that they do not affect the outcome of the research? The ORI did not have to prove that the data were material, but they did have to demonstrate motive in order to persuade DAB that someone had falsified data or intentionally misrepresented experimental procedures. It is difficult to show a motive for deliberately changing data when the changes have no effect on the conclusions or the probity of the paper.

PROBLEMS WITH MISCONDUCT INVESTIGATIONS

Some of the flaws in the way ORI handled this case occur also in committees impaneled by academic institutions to investigate allegations of scientific misconduct. One of the flaws was that the ORI scientific experts, or advisors, did not know the legal principles that they were supposed to apply in their investigation. Further, they did not really understand the science. (In the Popovic case they were not experts in the field of science involved: the isolation and propagation of a new retrovirus, so they did not understand the traditions of retrovirology on which Dr. Popovic based his approach to the problem of AIDS.) Moreover, they drew unreasonable inferences from the nonscientific evidence.

The process of dealing with allegations of scientific misconduct clearly must be improved. Committees at the university level need to better understand their charge, they need to better understand the applicable definitions, and they need to better understand how to conduct an investigation. Scientists do not automatically know how to conduct an investigation, how to weigh the evidence, and how to apply a standard of proof. They are used to doing statistical analyses according to established formulas, which is a very different matter.

In the meantime, we must be mindful of the costs involved. No one really knows yet how much it costs a university or an academic institution to conduct a scientific misconduct investigation. The cost to those who are accused is enormous. For 4 years Dr. Popovic suffered public humiliation. He was unable to practice his profession, he lost wages, and he incurred substantial legal fees. The loss to AIDS research, in my view, was incalculable. We must consider what all this means in terms of cost and decide whether what we are trying to protect is worth having a federal agency spend 4 years investigating trivial allegations having no effect on the integrity of the scientific literature.

ORI recently indicated that revisions to the definition of scientific misconduct will await the recommendations of a commission on research integrity, which is required by the recent NIH Reauthorization Act to study the problem yet again (PHS, 1993). The scientific community, which has a large stake in how this turns out, should participate fully in the regulatory process, because the definitions will be applied to all scientists for the foreseeable future.

It is also important for the scientific community to seek uniformity of regulations across government agencies. When the National Commission for the Protection of Human Subjects first looked at the regulations governing research involving human subjects (1974-1978), there were 26 different federal agencies that conducted or supported such research. The National Commission (1978) and the President's Commission for the Study of Ethical Problems in Medicine and Biomedical and Behavioral Research (1989) recommended that there be a uniform federal rule, so that review boards at academic institutions would not have to comply with 26 different sets of regulations. A uniform federal rule was finally adopted by the Office of Science and Technology Policy (1991). We very much need similar uniformity in the areas of scientific misconduct and conflicts of interest.

OWNERSHIP OF DATA

More and more frequently, I see cases that involve disagreements between scientists that really are not matters of scientific misconduct. Rather, they are issues of intellectual property, such as conflicts among members of a scientific team over authorship and access to data after members of the team relocate. For example, I recently represented a geneticist who worked with a clinical researcher on linkage studies to find a genetic basis for a certain disorder. The clinical researcher identified and examined the patients and their relatives, diagnosed those who had symptoms of the disorder and those who had the full-blown disease, and collected tissue samples. The geneticist then used tissue samples for his genetic research.

The geneticist and the clinical researcher had a falling out and, eventually, a parting of the ways. The clinical researcher then told the geneticist that he could not take any of the data with him when he left the institution. (Incidentally, the geneticist had done his part of the research under his own NIH grant, on which he was the principal investigator.) The clinician also told the geneticist that he could not be an author on any papers in the pipeline, even on papers reporting work they had done collaboratively before the team split up. The hardest part was that the geneticist was not permitted to have any of the data relevant to his own work, including immortalized cell lines, DNA, and computerized data analyses, which he himself had developed under his own NIH grant.

I have had other cases with similar controversies and conflicts over authorship and access to data. It is clear that academic institutions simply have not addressed this area, and they must do so. This is particularly important in dealing with science that has the potential for developing commercially valuable products.

When scientists work in an industrial setting, they normally sign employment contracts that spell out who has rights to the data they generate and what they may (or may not) do when they leave that particular company. There may even be noncompetition clauses. Academic scientists who are consultants for corporations also usually are asked to sign agreements spelling out their rights and responsibilities with respect to authorship, access to data, and rights to intellectual property.

There is no such analog in most academic institutions today, although a few have established guidelines. Harvard Medical School, for example, states clearly that primary data must remain in the laboratory where they were generated. The Johns Hopkins Medical School makes clear that a principal investigator may take primary data at the time of relocation but only with the written permission of the institution (because the data belong to the institution). NIH grants administration policies state that grantee institutions must maintain research-related records for a certain number of years (45 C.F.R. § 74.24). It is the institution, not the individual scientist, that is the recipient of the grant and is legally responsible to the funding agency for maintaining the data and ensuring compliance with applicable regulations. It is the institution, therefore, that must assert control over primary data. If controversies arise among members of a research team, the institution should step in and ensure that the data are treated properly.

Some medical institutions are beginning to train administrators in mediation to head off confrontations before they erupt into physical altercations in the surgical suite (Weiss, 1993). The same approach would be useful in academic laboratories to avoid allegations of scientific misconduct that arise from unresolved interpersonal conflicts.

GUIDELINES FOR ACADEMIA ON DATA AND AUTHORSHIP

Academic institutions should establish written policies making clear that research data belong to the institution, not to the individual scientist. They should add the general presumption that the data stay at the institution when a scientist leaves unless there is a written agreement to the contrary. Any such agreement should require that all of the collaborating scientists may have access to the data at any time. Of course, anyone leaving a research team should have copies of all data that are susceptible to copying. If the data cannot be copied, the departing scientist should have reasonable access to those data.

NIH takes the position that research funded by the federal government should be available to the people of the United States for their use (45 C.F.R. § 8.0). Accordingly, after any federally supported research has been published, the primary data and the biological materials should be available to all other scientists.

Where proprietary data or patentable ideas are involved, however, specific protections of intellectual property are appropriate. Policies designed for this purpose should be incorporated in the university's written policies and guidelines. Scientists should not be left to work out among themselves how to deal with potentially patentable ideas and materials when a team breaks up.

Universities should establish policies about authorship as well. The general rule should be that anyone who has substantially contributed to the design and conduct of a research project should be an author on a paper reporting that research, whether or not the person is still a member of the team when the paper is written and published. Deviations from the general rule could be negotiated and achieved with written permission from an appropriate university or institutional administrator, such as a vice president for research or a medical school dean.

INSTITUTIONAL REVIEW BOARDS AND RESEARCH ON HUMANS

An emerging question concerns what should happen if principal investigators misrepresent their research when they submit it to an institutional review board (IRB). The purpose of the IRB is to review research involving human subjects and to determine whether it is ethically acceptable (45 C.F.R. Part 46). IRBs decide what information must be provided to prospective research subjects, how the consent process should be accomplished, and how the consent forms should be worded. Violations of IRB requirements must be reported promptly to institutional officials and to funding agencies (45 C.F.R. § 46.103[b][5]). What is supposed to happen after that is not clear.

Several IRBs that have tried to initiate investigations into apparent violations of their requirements have been challenged by the accused scientists on due process grounds. In one case, a federal court made clear that an IRB is not a disciplinary body; it is a committee whose purpose under federal law is to protect human subjects (Halikas v. Minnesota, 1994). Thus, minimal due process is sufficient. What has not been worked out is the relationship among the IRB, the scientific misconduct regulations, and the institution's disciplinary policies and procedures. This area requires further discussion and clarification.

In the end, I hope we will achieve a uniform federal policy so that all federal agencies will adopt the same definitions and general principles, leaving to the individual academic institutions as much flexibility as possible to adopt the federal rules to their own needs, values, and procedures.

REFERENCES

Anderson, C. 1994. The aftermath of the Gallo case. Science 263:20-22.

Bivens, L. HHS News (Press Release, November 12, 1993) at 1-2.

Charrow, R. 1994. A novice's guide to jurisprudence: learning the law through ORI press releases. J. NIH Res. 6:64-66.

Re. Mikulas Popovic, M.D., Docket No. A-93-100, Decision No. 1446 (November 3,1993). Department of Health and Human Services, Department Appeals Board.

Halikas v. University of Minnesota, 856 F. Supp. 1331 (D. Minn. 1994).

National Commission for the Protection of Human Subjects. 1978. Pp. 14-17 in The Protection of Human Subjects in Research Conducted or Supported by Federal Agencies. Washington, D.C.: U.S. Government Printing Office.

National Institutes of Health (NIH). 1990. P. 15 in Guidelines for the conduct of research at the National Institutes of Health. Bethesda, Md.: NIH.

Office of Science and Technology Policy, Executive Office of the President. 1991. Federal policy for the protection of human subjects. Fed. Regist. 56:28002-28032.

Public Health Service (PHS). 1993. Establishment of Commission on Research Integrity. Fed. Regist. 58:66009

President's Commission for the Study of Ethical Problems in Medicine and Biomedical and Behavioral Research. 1989. First biennial report. Fed. Regist. 47:13272-13305.

Weiss, R. December 21, 1993. Doctors who fight over patients—literally. The Washington Post Health Magazine. P. 6.

16

Ethical Decision Making in a Pluralistic Society

DANIEL E. KOSHLAND, JR.

E thics is largely a matter of each person's independent judgment, because morality is largely defined by religion. Many religions have similar standards, but nevertheless, we have a pluralistic society with many religions. Thus, it is going to be very difficult for society to decide what is absolutely morally right and wrong. It is even more difficult to preemptively judge new scientific discoveries. Science has never been more powerful than it is today, and in the future it is going to be able to do a lot more things than it is going to be allowed to do.

Many scientists today feel perplexed by, and indignant about, the criticism of science. They think they have never done more for society and for its standard of living. In 1878, life expectancy was 34 years; in 1900, 47 years; in 1953, 67 years; and in 1991, 76 years. Scientists have added not only to life expectancy, but also to our pleasures in life. We have television and radio, which add to people's enjoyment. We have diminished mental illness and infectious diseases. So, with all of these amazing benefits, many scientists are perplexed about being criticized for the supposedly terrible damage that science has done to society.

Part of the reason for this criticism is that in a democracy we do not want to have any group that is adored as superior beings. The essence of a democracy is that any barber or taxi driver thinks he could run the country better than the president of the United States. We do not want people adoring a Hitler or a Mussolini and yet we ask people to acquire knowledge in some of these areas of science before they come to judgments. I was once interviewed by a television reporter who thought that scientists all got together every year and decided (against the wishes of humanity) what discoveries we were going to make and what research we would do. As we all know, that is not the way it is done. We cannot decide in advance what should and should not be discovered.

All knowledge is an advance. Two of the most controversial areas of knowledge—genetic engineering and cloning of organisms—are areas in which the advance of knowledge has been spectacular and has added to the increase in the life expectancy. Yet, even I, a strong proponent of science, see that there are some areas that we perhaps should avoid. However, in almost every case, I believe these areas are easily handled by society's decisions. It is up to scientists to inform the public of what they have done or are capable of doing and to give them the information in the most clear and simple terms. The public, in an informed dialogue, must decide what discoveries should be applied. It will be very dangerous if we start saying that there are certain areas of science that should not even be investigated.

So why are scientists criticized? Why are scientists accused of polluting the atmosphere? Why are we accused of doing these bad experiments in genetic engineering? A great deal of it is due to our successes. If the automobile had not been as popular as it is, we would not have the problem of clogged highways and carbon dioxide in the atmosphere. If people had not been living as long and so able to procreate, we would not have the overpopulation problem. People who criticize science do not pause to consider that the benefits of science have been the reasons for the excesses.

There is more to the public's reaction. A prescient book called *Future Shock* stated the essence of the problem: The rate of change in society is too rapid for us to assimilate. When golf was invented, it was a threat to the church. Suddenly, men had an alternative on Sunday mornings instead of going with the family to church. It was a serious problem, but gradually people coped with that problem and churches responded. Then the automobile came along, which was not merely a form of transportation, but also a change in the morality of society. In Victorian days, young girls did not go out with a man unless there was a chaperone present, but the automobile changed that and changed the morality of society. It took years for society to adjust to this new world. Then came birth control pills, surrogate mothers, and genetic engineering, all in rapid succession and following each other ever more rapidly. Society reacts: "These scientists are changing our lives." Not just a little bit, by inventing a television set you can turn on and off, but by changing moral values as well. Scientists must learn to assume responsibility for describing the ramifications and society must decide how far we should go. We do not want to stop the knowledge, but we want to consider the applications and their effects.

THE HUMAN GENOME PROJECT: IS IT BENEFICIAL?

Let us consider problems related to the Human Genome Project. One result of the project might be that we could do preemptive medicine, preventing problems before they become too extensive. There are people who say that we should not even know about the genome, that it is too much information and too predictive of the future. Long before the genome project, we knew about a disease called phenylketonuria, a genetic disease that could be predicted in a family if there were certain signs. This disease was likely to attack a young child, but if you eliminated phenylalanine from the child's diet in the early days of its life and controlled phenylalanine consumption later, that child was completely normal. If the child consumed the amount of phenylalanine that most babies usually consume, it would develop severe mental retardation and never become a fully functional adult. No one would seriously argue that you should deny the information to that family or that child. The Human Genome Project is really a big extension of this situation.

Another example is a disease called hypercholesterolemia. If you are homozygous for this disease, you produce cholesterol deficiencies such that you will get atherosclerosis at an early age and will probably be dead in your early teens. If you have a moderate version of the disease and are extraordinarily careful not to ingest any cholesterol, you could live to a reasonable age. There are many diseases that can be avoided by a change in lifestyle.

There can be positive aspects to knowing your genetic heritage. I happen to have been extraordinarily clever at picking my ancestors. I discovered recently that I can eat any amount of eggs Benedict and Hollandaise sauce without any damage to my arteries. I consider it terrible that I learned this just recently. If, because of the Human Genome Project, I had this information earlier, my life would have been much more enjoyable.

SOCIETAL PROBLEMS RELATING TO THE HUMAN GENOME PROJECT

What are the disadvantages of the genome project? Why would anybody say you should not know about the genome? Suppose a director of a medical school has access to an applicant's DNA sequence and sees that the applicant's life expectancy is low. Another applicant is almost as qualified and is going to live to be 80. What is the benefit for society of accepting people who are not going to be using their medical knowledge for very long instead of people who could use it for a long time? Should we be faced with that? A corporation, you could argue, wants to train young executives, and the longevity problem arises again. I believe that is a

194 / Ethics, Behavior, and Values in Science and Society

fairly easy problem to handle. Society as a whole must decide whether we are going to do that. There is a certain inefficiency in training M.D.s who will not get a chance to practice very long, but the alternative—telling young people that they have no future— is too terrible for us to contemplate and we are not going to do it. So we come to an understanding that life expectancy is not a prerequisite for medical school or other jobs.

The insurance problem, which is frequently mentioned as a result of the genome project, seems to me no problem at all. The insurance companies now have two forms of insurance. One is group insurance, which is what they generally like to sell because they sell to a large number of people, all of whom are getting insurance. They know ahead of time that some of those people are going to die or have very serious illness very quickly, but they use actuarial principles to figure that a certain number are going to be healthy and pay the premiums and a certain number are going to get sick.

There is no reason why genetic information is going to affect that. Insurance companies can use the same actuarial principles. Knowledge of the genome and medical science will only make it better for the insurance companies, because a certain number of diseases will be cured and those people will live longer than expected from past data.

But what about individual insurance? Insurance companies now ask very intrusive questions, such as Do you smoke? When did your brothers and sisters die? When did your parents die? When did your grandparents die? Have you had a heart attack? Have you refused any operations? In other words, they compile a lot of information and provide coverage on the basis of actuarial principles. There is no reason why DNA sequence cannot be one part of this body of information along with the rest.

Is that too intrusive? Maybe so. Laws can make it illegal to have insurance companies get that information, but all it will change is the actuarial calculations. It is not either moral or immoral. It is society's decision that, in effect, fairly healthy people will pay a little higher rates to cover people who have less life expectancy. However, there is a reciprocal requirement. If the insurance company should not have that DNA information, individuals who want to be insured also should not have it. If you allowed people access to that information and they knew they were going to die soon, they could then buy millions of dollars of insurance and tilt the actuarial tables. So when people consider the morality of insurance, they must also consider the reciprocal obligations of all concerned.

The genome project is a blessing. It is going to save many lives. The information from the project is already enormously valuable. We have now found, for example, that an inheritable disease such as colorectal cancer is related to other cancers, such as kidney cancer and uterine cancer. They are all related by the same genes. That means if you have a family history of any of these cancers, you should have a colonoscopy. Colorectal cancer is a 100 percent curable disease if you are warned in time. If you do not have the genetic tendency, your statistics are lower and you can avoid the rather unpleasant colonoscopy.

That kind of information is going to be available with DNA sequencing, and I see very little reason not to go ahead with it. You can make various rules about using DNA information for jobs and insurance, but with insurance, you are just changing actuarial calculations. I was amused in the discussion on health care that some people were outraged that the insurance companies were actually turning people down because they already had a disease. Insurance was seen as sort of a civil right that you cannot be denied. In other words, after you have cancer you go and take out insurance, or after you become pregnant you take out insurance for health care for pregnant mothers. There is nothing moral in that. If you could be allowed to get insurance after you know you have the disease, it would be a wonderful system, but you would have to pay quite different premiums. The actuarial system depends on a number of healthy people carrying the load for people who are ill.

CLONING

What about cloning individuals? I am more hesitant here. My initial reaction was that nobody should be cloned. Then I thought of having eight people exactly like me and all of us on the Supreme Court. Then I began to think the Celtics would probably like five people just like Larry Bird and the Lakers five just like Magic Johnson. Would that be a good idea? You could get Secretariats produced in large numbers and horse races would become a thing of the past. So I think there is some limit on this.

However, there does not seem to be an absolute disadvantage to cloning. The initial reaction of most people is that you cannot use humans for experiments, but that is modified in ethical drug trials. The National Institutes of Health, for example, makes it difficult to change the germ line. That really is peculiar because we are changing the germ line all the time. Insulin is used to keep alive people with diabetes who formerly would have died very early in life. That is changing the germ line enormously. We are keeping very ill people alive and are changing the germ line for the worse. Now, if someone wants to help a family who has had diabetes in its germ line for years and years by putting in a good gene so the next generations will not have that problem, is that a terrible thing?

I am defective person. My eyes are such that I was 20/200 when I was a kid. I would not have seen a saber tooth tiger until it came up to lick my face, so my family and all of its descendants would have been done for. I wear glasses to correct that defect. We do not have fur so we live in air conditioned rooms and wear clothes. So the idea of keeping defective people alive is something society has been doing for a long time, but all of a sudden it is a bad thing to change the germ line. I am not sure that I understand this logic.

Genetic engineering can be abused. I do not want to understate this. However, if a child has diabetes, you ask to correct the gene. Everybody would say that is fine. If a child has an IQ of 50, or the family has the gene for an IQ of 50, we would all probably agree that the gene should be corrected. What about a family that has a series of children who have IQs of 95 and they would like to have children with IQs of 120? The children would get into Harvard and do very well in some law school. Is that bad? You start worrying a little about that.

Once you invent something people are going to want to use it; I do not want to pretend that a discovery in science will not be used in some bad ways. Consider again the cloning of humans. Suppose you could produce 20 identical people who could solve a very important problem by being part of an experiment on why violence exists. If these 20 identical cloned people were to grow up in 20 different environments with good homes, bad homes, ghettos, and very aggressive communities, how would that change their lives? Would it be a terrible thing to use cloning for that purpose?

EXPERIMENTING WITH HUMANS

We are already experimenting with humans in major ways without knowing it. We pass laws that constrain our behavior, and we are not always sure that it is going to turn out correctly. So it seems to me that each of these decisions is going to have to be decided not on a moral or ethical basis, but on the basis of common sense. I think we all have sort of an ingrained sense of what is right and wrong, but sometimes in the modern world of television and instant slogans we get the wrong impression.

Several years ago I was asked to discuss the question of whether or not we should work with microcephalic children. This is a "child" born without a brain. The brain essentially begins at the end of the stem, so the child really has no brain. In the old days it would have died very, very quickly, but now it can be kept alive on a life support system. I would not call this "a person" because the courts have decided that death occurs when the brain goes dead. So this organism, if you want to call it that, has no brain, yet it is functioning. Its heart is functioning so it can be kept alive. Some people were suggesting using its organs for organ transplants or using it for the study of development. My advice was that you might learn a lot of science, but it would be too ghoulish. People would react against scientists. Recently a federal judge ruled that a family who had a microcephalic baby and who wanted to end the life support system would not be allowed to do so because it violated the rights of that so-called child.

I think it is rather interesting that a group of scientists decided it was too ghoulish to run experiments or keep children alive for organs that could be used later, and yet a judge sees it from a different point of view. He cites the rights of children and orders this family to do a very expensive procedure in a situation where this organism will never develop into what anyone would call a child.

The same situation arose in California recently where the growth hormone made by recombinant DNA, which produces much more milk in cows by genetic engineering methods, has been declared a terrible thing. It is an amusing case because although the Food and Drug Administration (FDA) said that the product is not dangerous to people's health, it was pressured by dairy farmers to say use of the hormone would produce so much milk that the price of milk would drop, and therefore the hormone should be banned. The FDA finally came out for use of the growth hormone but did so with much hesitation. This was noted by the people who are against it and they waged a big campaign. Moreover, the California law is rather interesting. The law says supermarkets have to say that this milk is guaranteed not to have this hormone, which is a natural hormone. All the genetic engineering has done is to produce more of it in cows. So if this law is passed, it means that no milk can be sold in California because the milk contains natural hormone. California already is a nuclear-free zone. It is now also going to be a milk-free zone.

NEED FOR PUBLIC EDUCATION

There is great pressure on scientists to be perfect. However, for all future experiments to be ethically correct requires a concomitant commitment on the part of the public, and in particular the media, to have a reasonable amount of scientific information so that they can make informed judgments about scientific matters. Scientists do not have to explain to the public the details of DNA or the structure of a protein before they can get an opinion on whether fertilizing eggs in a test tube for childless couples is approved, but society needs to make the decisions: Do we want to have this technology used? Do we want to use it under certain limited circumstances?

Scientists have a big advantage over other people in helping society solve these problems because scientists have experience with complexity. They are used to dealing with complicated issues that are not clear-cut. I happen to be in the pro-choice group on abortion, but I was not pleased with the people who argued that pro-choice was simply morally right and a woman had the right to her own body. Good slogan, but oversimplified. There were many devout Catholics who were also good friends of mine who really felt that it was morally wrong. That is an illustration of what I mentioned earlier. In a pluralistic society there are going to be people with deep religious convictions, so no one can say what is morally right for everyone. There have to be compromises. Each person has a choice on that issue. Some of the people who said a woman has control of her own body as an argument for abortion then reverted to the other side on surrogate motherhood, saying a woman should not be allowed to have a child for something as crass as money. If a woman has the right to her own body, she should have the right to create life as well as a right to destroy it.

Many of these issues are very complicated and will require a great deal of common sense, but the decision making is going to be made easier by people who understand complexity. We need to sort things out in the very big mixture of things rather than just state a big moral principle and be stuck with this generalization.

Many of these subjects are not clear-cut morally or ethically. When recombinant DNA research began, nobody could have predicted the big biotechnology industry, how valuable it would be, how many lives it would save, how many jobs it would create. We now have an enormous capacity to solve a lot of problems. A good example of a benefit of the Human Genome Project is that it will be particularly useful for multigenic diseases, for example, mental illness. It has been estimated that 50 percent of the people who are homeless are mentally ill. So when the president of the United States says he is going to solve the homeless problem by retraining, somebody has not told him what the real problem is. If you can solve the problem of mental illness indirectly by a genome project, it seems to me that you have contributed an enormous amount to society.

We, scientists and nonscientists, are all going to have to work together. I think that scientists who are in the ivory tower would much rather just solve scientific problems. Earlier in my life, I said that my job was to solve problems. Society could use the science it wanted and I should not be forced to get out of my laboratory and explain to other people what was going on. I now think that is impossible. Discoveries in science are now so powerful that we are affecting people's lives every day. We are going to have to explain the nature of these problems, the nature of discoveries, and the random nature of investigator-initiated research, which I think brought us to where we are today.

Some discoveries are going to be made that will have a big effect on society, and society has a right to hear about these discoveries. It is going to be a lot of work for all of us, but that is the way that the ethical problems need to be solved.

17

Ethical Issues Surrounding the New Technology as Applied to Health Care

MARK A. ROTHSTEIN

One way of looking at the advances that have been made in molecular genetics over the past decade is to look at increasingly smaller molecular units. That is, we can go from examining at the level of cells to the nuclei, chromosomes, genes, and individual nucleotide base pairs. What I would like to do is to back up: to look, not at such a small piece of the puzzle, but at the level of the individual, the family, the group, and, indeed, society.

When Dr. James D. Watson began his tenure as director of the National Center for Human Genome Research in 1991, he committed at least 3 percent of the budget to the study of ethical, legal, and social implications of the project (Cook-Deegan, 1994). Now we are up to 5 percent. It was not clear to many people then what the ethical, legal, and social implications would be, but Watson had great foresight and recognized that new discoveries in the field of genetics would raise a variety of issues. This certainly has proven to be the case. I will cover some of the issues identified by the Human Genome Project and then focus on one particular aspect of the ethical problems or issues raised by the new genetics, namely the effect on health care and reproduction.

ETHICAL, LEGAL AND SOCIAL IMPLICATIONS PROGRAM

The Ethical, Legal and Social Implications Program (ELSI) of the Human Genome Project conducts ongoing research on such areas as the organization and dynamics of research, intellectual property issues, technology transfer, commercialization, and human subjects research (Table 17-1). ELSI also addresses clinical practice issues, many of which have yet to be explored. They involve questions such as when a technology is ready to go from the laboratory to the clinical practice setting and include diagnostic technologies as well as gene therapy (Institute of Medicine, 1994).

There are also a range of public health issues raised by ELSI. For example, what decisions must be made about allocating funding for genome research and genetic services? There are also privacy issues raised by the accumulation of DNA information in data banks for forensic and other purposes. What is genetic privacy? How does it apply between the individual and the government or among individuals within a given family setting? We also have a very wide range of civil rights issues raised by the Human Genome Project. Can employers perform genetic tests them-

TABLE 17-1   Research Agenda for the Ethical, Legal and Social Implications Program of the Human Genome Project

Science Policy Issues
    Organization and dynamics of genomic research
    Intellectual property policy
    Commercialization practices
    Human subjects research rules
Clinical Practice Issues
    Technology assessment criteria
    When and who to test
    Information disclosure practices
    Counseling practices
Health Policy Issues
    Public health role of genetic services
    Allocation of resources to genetic services
Privacy Issues
    DNA databanking policies
    DNA identification standards
    Legal definitions of "genetic privacy"
    Intra-familial communication issues
Civil Rights Issues
    Employment testing policies
    Health insurance underwriting practices
    Life and disability insurance
    Social discrimination/stigmatization
    Genetics and racism
Educational Policy Issues
    Clinical education models
    Public education models
    Health professional training

selves? Can they gain access to genetic test results obtained by the individual in the clinical setting? Can health insurance companies, life insurance companies, or disability insurance companies see the information? Anyone with a stake in the future health status of an individual might well want to gain access to genetic test results so they can calculate the future expense they may have to bear for that person. Is this information confidential?

To what extent will the accumulation of genetic information increase the stigma on individuals who are currently affected or who may be affected in the future (their family members and others)? What is the prospect for eugenics? It was not that long ago that there was a major eugenics movement in the United States that we exported, unfortunately, to Nazi Germany in the 1930s, which led to tremendous horror, as we all know. Finally, what educational needs does the Human Genome Project present? Will we need to upgrade professional education, public education, and the education of particular groups that need to know about advances in genetics? We are way behind in that area as well. From these broad questions, I have selected 10 specific questions that give a sense of the unanswerable nature of the issues raised by human genome research.

QUESTIONS ILLUSTRATING THE UNANSWERABLE NATURE OF THE ISSUES

1. If access to prenatal genetic testing (and abortion) is limited to affluent people, then poor people will bear a disproportionate burden of genetic disease. Is this fair? What are the social consequences?

The Supreme Court continues to uphold the Roe v. Wade decision of 1973 (*Roe v. Wade*, 1973). However, one of the major impediments to actually obtaining an abortion is that public funding for abortion is greatly limited in many areas. If we limit prenatal genetic testing and abortion of affected fetuses to the wealthy or the well insured, what is the societal implication? What will it mean to society if substantially all of the children born with serious genetic defects over the next decade or two are born to uninsured, underinsured, and indigent people? What does that mean in terms of society's view of these diseases? It is bad enough to have the disease and to have the stigma associated with the disease, but the diseases will not only be terrible genetic diseases, they will be terrible genetic diseases of the poor.

What effect will that have on our willingness to expend dollars for research to cure these diseases, for treatment of these individuals, for rehabilitation services, and for special education? These are issues we should confront, and they are not hypothetical issues. The way a questions is framed often determines the answer. For example, today, if the drug abuse problem is seen as a problem of the suburbs and the middle class, the solution to drug abuse is treatment. If drug abuse is seen as a problem of the underclass, the solution is the criminal justice system.

2. If genetic "enhancement" (for example, height or intelligence) became available in the future, would rich people be tall and smart and poor people short and stupid?

If genetic enhancement becomes available, it does not take too much imagination to assume that it would not be universally available. Suppose we could increase height and intelligence through various means. Does that mean that rich people would be tall and smart and poor people would be short and stupid? This, it seems to me, is social Darwinism leading to biological Darwinism (Miller, 1994).

3. If we allow parents, through either preimplantation genetic testing or prenatal genetic testing and abortion, to select against certain conditions, such as spina bifida and Down syndrome, is this tantamount to saying that people already affected with these conditions have less value?

If we allow parents to select against certain conditions, what does that say to people who are already affected with the conditions? This is an issue that greatly concerns those in the disability rights community because some have charged that we are essentially trying to wipe out people like them. They believe we are making a statement that their lives are not as valued as ours (Kaplan, 1994). I disagree with that for various reasons, but I think you can see the line of reasoning. We have to consider not just how to avoid the birth of people with certain conditions, but also how to deal with those conditions as they exist in people and how to treat these people differently, perhaps, from the way we now treat them.

4. What new psychological burdens will genetic testing place on parents and children, and what effect will new genetic information have on relationships?

Dr. Nancy Wexler tells the story of a woman who said that she wanted her two minor children tested for Huntington disease because she only had enough money to send one to Harvard (Wexler, 1992). That strikes me as the dark side of genetic testing. Genetic testing is certainly very valuable, but what effects will it have on families? What problems are raised by testing for recessive disorders? Parents often do not properly understand what it means to be a carrier of a recessive disorder. Many studies show that these children have been stigmatized by their parents, siblings, and peers. They are not allowed to climb trees or play football or ride bikes because their parents view them as more vulnerable, obviously because of inadequate counseling and education (Clayton, 1992).

5. Will an increasing emphasis on health care cost containment create eugenic pressures?

Is this likely to arise? I am somewhat optimistic that we are not going to have the master race syndrome of eugenics, that is, positive eugenics. However, I am very troubled by the prospect that an emphasis on health care cost containment could lead to negative eugenics and pressures to avoid the birth of children who will become high-cost users of the health care system.

We have ample illustrations of this actually taking place. Suppose a child is born with a fatal, incurable childhood genetic disorder. The child lives for a year or two and costs $500,000 or $1 million to treat. Now the mother is pregnant with another child. The family has no private or government-paid insurance, and the second child will be affected by the disorder. Then the mother has a third child and a fourth and a fifth. At some point, is someone in the country going to say, "For $1 million we can vaccinate X number of children. For $1 million we can perform surgeries on X number of people. For $1 million we can do all these other public health functions. We cannot afford as a society to invest $1 million and another million and another million on these people." Are we going to prevent this woman from having any more children? If so, how? Through compulsory sterilization? Through compulsory abortion? Through compulsory birth control? I think that even if there is a low likelihood of something like that occurring, the prospect of it and the size of the disruption to society demands that we start thinking about such situations.

6. Are special concerns raised if we discover genes related to behavioral traits such as alcoholism, intelligence, homosexuality, or violent behavior?

In Colorado there already is a program for fragile X syndrome that screens individuals who have already been identified by their teachers in special education classes (Webb, 1993). Suppose we find a gene or genes for alcoholism. Does that mean we are going to be more—or less—sympathetic to alcoholics? One could argue that we ought to be more sympathetic because we would realize that they had no control over their genetic makeup. However, there would be some who would say, "Why did you start drinking, knowing you carried the gene for alcoholism?" The same thing is true for other conditions (Brock, 1992).

There are school systems in this country that are anxious to embark on screening programs for learning disabilities. Schools could then place students into certain educational programs, but in doing so they may disregard whether there is evidence that they need specialized instruction and the social stigma that goes along with identification as learning disabled.

7. Is genetic information different from other medical information? If so, what special measures are needed to protect confidentiality?

In insurance, employment, and some other areas, it is difficult, in theory, to make a case that genetic information or genetic conditions are different from other conditions (NIH-DOE, 1993). If you have a neurological disorder, for example, what the disease is and how it came about is seemingly irrelevant to your right to treatment. However, genetic information may in some cases be treated differently, because if I am affected, my children, my parents, and my siblings may be affected. A condition that is vertically transmissible may have a great deal of stigma attached to it. It may be a condition that by its genetic nature tends to run more frequently in certain ethnic or racial groups. For many reasons, when we are confronted with genetic information we have to be even more vigilant in protecting the confidentiality of this medical information. The question is raised, of course, how do you do that? The answer is not clear to me or anyone else at the moment.

8. Are health care providers, consumers, the media, and the public prepared for the vast increase in genetic information?

The answer is no in all these categories. First of all, we have only 1,000 or fewer medical geneticists in this country. If and when we develop multiplex genetic testing that can be done in the doctor's office, it is going to be done in the office of the primary care physician. That physician may have gone to medical school 25 years ago when none of this genetic information was available. What kinds of continuing medical education programs are we going to have? Who is going to do the genetic counseling that is so essential when you tell people of their risk for certain disorders or their likelihood of certain disorders? If we wait until the clinical setting, when someone walks into the office, it is going to be too late. The issues are so complicated that it may be too difficult to explain during that visit, for example, the difference between recessive and X-linked traits. That is why we are embarking on an aggressive program of teaching high school students the basics of the new genetics, including the ethical, legal, and social implications: when people come in for treatment, they will be already a step ahead in understanding their diagnosis and analysis (Andrews et al., 1994).

Media efforts in this area have been disappointing. I have seen too many television shows that try to deal with all the scientific issues as well as all the ethical issues in 30 minutes. Even knowing what they are trying to do, I still do not understand what they are saying. I pity the public that must be incredibly confused by all this information. We need to break down the information into meaningful portions and devise some way of getting the public interested in these issues. We also need to demonstrate to the print and electronic media that the public has a longer attention span than 15 seconds. Until we do that, the media will not produce programming or articles that go into the necessary depth of analysis.

9. *Is it reasonable to spend $3 billion on the Human Genome Project, which initially may benefit relatively few people, when much of the developing world lacks minimum health standards (e.g., nutrition, sanitation, and vaccinations) and when millions of Americans lack access to basic health services?*

Scientists and consumers have questioned the genome project from the perspective of cost. Why should we spend all that money on this project and not on something else? Arguably, we would save many more lives if we cleaned up the water supply and provided basic access to health care, but that is a somewhat short-sighted view. With the information from the genome project, we are not only going to treat people with exotic disorders, but we are also going to be able to identify people at increased risk of common diseases, such as breast cancer, colon cancer, and heart disease. What we learn in the genetics field is going to have great application elsewhere.

10. *In what ways will genetics affect our culture? Will genetic-based reductionism and determinism dominate individual and collective thought in the next century?*

Will we as a society be overcome by this genetic information? Will we embrace reductionism, that is, will we focus only on the genetic component of a problem? Will we subscribe to determinism (our destiny is in our genes, my lot is cast)? What are the implications of that? For example, will we become a society of risk takers? "I'm carrying the gene for these three or four things, so I'll start sky diving, scuba diving, driving a race car, or wrestling alligators, and why not? I have nothing to lose." We could become a society of paranoids, the "worried well," concerned about conditions for which we may have a statistically increased but still small risk of developing. Will we become a society where people think every cough is the first sign of lung cancer and every accidentally dropped paper clip is the first sign of a neurological disorder? Will half of us be paranoid and the other half too busy sky diving to worry about it? How will these two groups interact?

ADDRESSING ISSUES IN THE SHORT TERM

From these very difficult questions we could conclude that the technology itself is undesirable. Maybe we should stop or limit the technology so that these problems will disappear. However, the technology itself is not the problem. I recently read a very appropriate quotation from, of all people, C. S. Lewis, who said, "Man's power over nature turns out to be a power exercised by some men over other men with nature as its instrument." It is not the technology that is going to cause eugenics. It is not the technology that is going to cause intrafamilial problems and discrimination. It is all of us, if we let it. We must be extremely watchful to ensure that all of these issues and many others will be considered along with the new experiments and the exciting developments in treatment.

Let me suggest some ways in which I believe these issues can and should be addressed in the short term. I have six suggestions that I think we should consider in the health care reform debate:

• Make appropriate genetic services available to all. The key word, of course, is appropriate. We do not want to embark on a population-wide carrier screening program for every imaginable disorder. That would be a tremendous waste of resources; services such as pre-symptomatic genetic testing for those at risk would be appropriate. In the health care reform proposals debated by Congress in 1994, there were no specific provisions for the coverage of genetic services.

• Safeguard autonomy in reproduction. We have to be very careful not to allow any sort of direct or indirect coercion to influence individuals' reproductive decision making. People should have autonomy to make these difficult choices.

• Expand professional and public education programs.

• Prohibit genetic discrimination by health insurers. We should prevent genetic discrimination by prohibiting health insurers from denying coverage on the basis of preexisting conditions or on the basis of having a particular genotype.

• Prohibit genetic discrimination by employers. Under any version of health care reform, employers will continue to play a crucial role. Today, 80 percent of employers with 1,000 or more employees are self-insured. A self-insured employer bears the risk of illness and associated health care costs directly, dollar for dollar. Because in any given year 5 percent of health care claimants represent 50 percent of the health care dollars, there is a tremendous incentive to weed out a small group of very-high-cost users. If we prohibit health insurance companies from discriminating on the basis of genetic traits, we may be simply shifting the level of discrimination from the insurance company to employers. That will be doubly detrimental, because not only will people be denied insurance coverage, they also will be denied jobs. So we will have created a whole class of people who are unemployable. They may never become ill; they may simply be at an increased risk that someone considers to be unacceptably high.

• Protect the confidentiality of genetic information. When bills on medical privacy in general are introduced, genetic issues and genetic confidentiality must be considered.

I do not want to dampen enthusiasm for the new genetic technology—it is brilliant and exciting—but I am suggesting that many very complicated legal, ethical, social, moral, and societal issues need to be worked out. The time to work these out or to begin to work them out is now, not in the year 2010. We have legislation pending. We do not want to go down the wrong path. If we adopt these six measures that I have suggested, I think that would certainly point us in the right direction. Then, perhaps, we could take on those 10 even more difficult social issues presented earlier.

REFERENCES

Andrews, L. B., J. E. Fullerton, N. A. Holtzman, and A. E. Motulsky, eds. 1994. Assessing Genetic Risks: Implications for Health and Social Policy, ch. 5, Public Education in Genetics. Washington, D.C.: National Academy Press.

Brock, D. W. 1992. The Human Genome Project and human identity. Houston Law Rev. 29:7-22.

Clayton, E. W. 1992. Screening and treatment of newborns. Houston Law Rev. 29:85-148.

Cook-Deegan, R. 1994. The Gene Wars. New York: W.W. Norton.

Institute of Medicine. 1994. Assessing Genetic Risks: Implications for Health and Social Policy. Washington, D.C.: National Academy Press.

Kaplan, D. 1994. Prenatal screening and diagnosis: the impact on persons with disabilities, women & prenatal testing. Pp. 49-61 in Women and Prenatal Testing: Facing the Challenges of Genetic Technology, K. H. Rothenberg and E. J. Thomson, eds. Columbus, Ohio: Ohio State University Press.

Miller, H. I. 1994. Gene therapy for enhancement. Lancet 344:316-317.

NIH-DOE Working Group on Ethical, Legal, and Social Implications of Human Genome Research, Genetic Information and Health Insurance. 1993. Report of the Task Force on Genetic Information and Insurance. Washington, D.C.: National Institutes of Health.

Roe v. Wade, 410 U.S. 113 (1973).

Webb, J. 1993. A fragile case for screening? New Scientist 140:1905-1906.

Wexler, N. 1992. Clairvoyance and caution: repercussions from the Human Genome Project. Pp. 211-243 in The Code of Codes, D. J. Kevles and L. Hood, eds. Cambridge, Mass.: Harvard University Press.

18

Biotechnology Applications and Women's Health Issues

RUTH ELLEN BULGER

W e are entering a scientific revolution that has enormous potential to bring about change in the health care that Americans
receive. Drug or cell therapy will be specifically targeted to the
precise molecular or cellular defect. The ability to keep patients alive will
continue to expand as will the ability to accomplish new procedures.

We are also in a rapidly changing time in relation to the application of
biotechnology to issues of women's health. Several reasons underlie this
changing scene. It has become evident that health advantages accrue to
subgroups of people who are used as subjects in clinical trials. Yet recent
news reports have repeatedly publicized the fact that women have not
been included as subjects in the study population of certain large-scale
prevention trials. Such trials include the Physician's Health Study of 1989,
which evaluated the role of aspirin in the prevention of heart attacks; the
Multiple Risk Factor Intervention Trial in 1977, which investigated the
relationships among life-style factors, cholesterol levels, and heart disease; and the Baltimore Longitudinal Study, which did not include women
until its 20th year (Multiple Risk Factor Intervention Trial Group, 1977;
Steering Committee of the Physician Health Study Research Group, 1989).

In addition, women have been shown to be treated less aggressively
than men for certain medical conditions. Khan et al. (1990) found that
differences in preoperative functional class (e.g., later referral for coronary bypass surgery) and greater age, rather than sex, account for the
higher operative mortality of women in coronary bypass surgery. Tobin
et al. (1987) had earlier shown that even with abnormal exercise test re-

sults, only 4 percent of women with chest pain were referred for coronary arteriography whereas 40 percent of men were referred.

In the area of human immunodeficiency virus (HIV), Minkoff and DeHovitz (1991) found that little was known about the natural course of HIV infection in women. Recently, women and adolescent girls infected with HIV were shown to get fewer medications and have fewer hospital admissions (20 percent fewer) and outpatient visits than did comparably sick men (Hellinger, 1993).

Although the extent of and precise populations comprising what has been referred to as the underrepresentation of women as subjects of research has not been well documented (Institute of Medicine, 1994), the oft-repeated reports cited above have played an important role in galvanizing women into action. Women are no longer sitting back passively and accepting what the research and health care systems offer for their needs. Instead, women are asking questions, assessing assumptions, and working together to ensure that their concerns are being addressed.

How did we get into this situation of inequity concerning the participation of women in clinical research and, hence, the usefulness of the research results to the care of women who are ill? I believe that modern science has been operating with a series of colored lenses over scientists' collective eyes, distorting our view and leaving us viewing clinical trials "through a glass darkly." As we progress through the postmodern era, we are recognizing that these lenses exist and are removing them from our eyes so that we can see more clearly, but how to navigate in this new terrain remains problematic. Many of these lenses relate to how technology has been applied to men and women.

LENS 1: SCIENCE IS OBJECTIVE

Thomas Kuhn (1970) said in his book *The Structure of Scientific Revolution*, "The early developmental stages of most sciences have been characterized by continual competition between a number of distinct views of nature . . . all roughly compatible with the dictates of scientific observation and method. What differentiated these various schools was not one or another failure of method—they were all scientific—but what we shall come to call their incommensurable ways of seeing the world and of practicing science in it. . . . An apparently arbitrary element, compounded of personal and historical accident, is always a formative ingredient of the beliefs espoused by a given scientific community at a given time."

Or as James Miller (1989) describes the postmodern world, "The world is understood to be relative, indeterminate, and participatory. Contemporary physics, however, has effectively shown that while there can be a relative objectivity in the practice of science . . . there is no observation in which the object observed and the subject observing are absolutely separate. That is to say, there are no 'facts' in nature independent of some particular observer. . . . All knowers are participants in that which is to be known."

Removing lens 1 will help us separate issues of scientific validity and methodology from underlying questions and beliefs about social and ethical values that are embedded within our seemingly objective scientific endeavors. Many of the lenses discussed below are, in fact, examples of the confusion of subjective viewpoints with scientific fact.

LENS 2: THE APPLICATION OF BIOMEDICAL DEVELOPMENT LEADS TO CONTINUOUS PROGRESS

John Dominic Crossan (1988), in comparing progress with change in art and science finds that one great Western claim is that there is past and future progress of the human race. Evolution has not been a neutral word denoting change, but a positive word implying improvement. He argues that the history of art shows no evolutionary progress across the centuries. "Therefore, we have movement without progress, we have change without improvement. This does not mean that at any given moment there may not be good or bad, better or worse, in art but that if one tried to make a graph of its history, over the centuries, the graph would look, I suppose, rather like a person's electrocardiogram. lt would not be a clear, rising line, but neither would it be a circle closed in on itself. The question, then, is whether such a graph might not be a master paradigm for all human activities, not just art."

He continues, "Our science, precisely as science, is not better than neolithic science. It is simply different. If one insists that modern science is both different and better, it might be as well to remember that the bill for modern science has not yet been paid in full. We do know that neolithic science did not destroy the earth or render its climate unlivable. So let us settle for difference rather than progress between neolithic and modern science, and let us hope we are as creative as humans then were, and at no greater cost to our humanity or the earth's well-being."

Questions that we might ask that would help us recognize change versus progress include: Do applications of the new biotechnology to people really improve the health of the individual (e.g., does it work)? In applying the technology to the individual, what social, legal, ethical, and economic quandaries do we cause in the person's life or community?

Consider some examples of applications of technology to women's health care that show change but not progress. Electronic fetal monitoring was developed to detect fetal asphyxia and is now used routinely in most deliveries. The 1989 Institute of Medicine (IOM) report entitled *Medical Professional Liability and the Delivery of Obstetrical Care* discusses the history of the use of electronic fetal monitoring. The report shows that the technology was not adequately evaluated before its use became widespread. It was never formally evaluated by the Food and Drug Administration because it was in use before the enactment of the Medical Devices Act of 1976 (P.L. 94-295). The overwhelming data from later evaluations of this technology, including nine randomized clinical trials, show little or no benefit to its use in reducing neonatal mortality and morbidity. Most cases of brain damage are not due to delivery events, the frequency of most forms of brain damage has not decreased with widespread use of electronic fetal monitoring, and the causes of most cerebral palsy and mental retardation are still not known.

A second example of a change in the use of technology that was not necessarily an advance is earlier diagnosis for various medical conditions. Black and Welch (1993) maintain that by the use of a panoply of new diagnostic techniques, such as computed tomography, magnetic resonance imaging, and ultrasonography, minute abnormalities can be detected well before they produce any clinical signs or symptoms. In fact, we may well be detecting a broader spectrum of change or disease whose natural history and response to interventions are unknown. These authors claim that we could be labeling patients with a disease that they do not have and giving them therapy that they do not need. This early diagnosis may explain why certain diseases now appear to be epidemic.

An example used by Black and Welch is the early diagnosis of breast cancer. With the lower detection threshold for this disease produced by the use of modern technology, we have moved from looking at a suspicious mass to looking at a suspicious microcalcification. If we are identifying a lesion earlier, then a new test or a new treatment given in this early stage will appear falsely to prolong survival when compared with historical controls. Bias also results because the probability that disease will be detected by testing is directly proportional to the length of its detectable preclinical phase, which is inversely related to the rate of progression. Therefore, disease detected by testing tends to progress less rapidly than disease that would ultimately present clinically in the absence of testing. The authors believe that an identified lesion may be a pseudodisease that might regress, remain stable, or progress too slowly to be clinically apparent in the patient's life. This becomes an issue of extreme importance to women that can only definitively be decided by clinical trials involving women. We need to ensure that new technologies are well tested before diffusion into practice and that side effects are identified before use.

LENS 3: THE DOCTOR KNOWS BEST

With the growth of various rights movements (e.g., civil rights, women's rights, and gay and lesbian rights) and the decrease in shared value systems in modern society, the traditional paternalistic model of health care is being replaced by a model of patient participation in decision making. Many patients now wish to be educated and empowered to make medical decisions for themselves. This desire, of course, varies with the patient. Some patients still want the doctor to make decisions, others want to be a part of the decision-making process, whereas others want to make the decisions by themselves.

However, doctors can and do affect patient choices. For example, Lurie et al. (1993) showed that the sex of the physician treating the patient affects the care given. For example, women are more likely to undergo screening with Pap smears and mammograms if the physician is a woman rather than a man.

A patient's role in the decision-making process is especially important when a patient's preferences would affect the treatment chosen or when a patient, perhaps being more risk averse, might weigh the risks and benefits differently from how the doctor might weigh them. Such a process includes the patient's personal evaluation of quality-of-life issues as part of decision making.

One approach to facilitate the inclusion of patients in the decision-making process is the production of a series of interactive video programs by the nonprofit Foundation for Informed Medical Decision Making, created by Albert Mulley, Jr., and John Wennberg (Randall, 1993). Two of their programs relate to breast cancer: the first examines the choice of the kind of surgery to be done and the second looks at the use of adjuvant therapy in treatment. Interactive videos are especially useful when choices are affected by patients' values and preferences. Women have been leaders in wanting to be part of medical decisions concerning their own lives.

LENS 4: ADULT WHITE MALES ARE THE NORM

The preferential use of adult white males as the traditional (and as we have discussed earlier, sometimes the only) subjects for clinical studies was not based on any thought-out belief that the health of males was more worthy or important but on the unexamined belief that the data obtained could be generalized to other groups. Only with the recognition and testing of this belief was the lack of uniformity of response by sex, race, and ethnicity able to be appreciated. The full extent of the real differences in the way women and men and members of various ethnic and racial groups differ with respect to drug pharmacokinetics and pharmaco-dynamics is presently unknown. Excluding women from participation in trials limits the physician's ability to treat diseases in women.

Because few comprehensive data exist on differences between male and female responses to drug treatments, one provision of the National Institutes of Health Revitalization Act of 1993 (P.L. 103-43) is a requirement to create a registry focused on collecting women's health data. Although such data are needed, the registry that has been proposed is much too narrow; such a registry would be much more meaningful if it included data from men and women from various racial and ethnic groups. This more complete database would be useful in development of a research agenda.

The recently released IOM (1994) report entitled *Women and Health Research* provides data on this topic. It finds that, fortunately, in most situations assessed so far, men and women do not react differently to diseases and treatments if data are normalized for factors such as body size; therefore including both sexes in trials is reasonable because treatment effects should not differ. However, the medical literature describes various differences in the physiological and psychosocial responses of women and men to medical interventions. When there are, or there are valid reasons to believe there might be, differences between the sexes regarding the treatment being investigated, then it would make sense to include both sexes in trials and in sufficient numbers to test for sex differences.

The considerations discussed regarding women also apply to the inclusion in trials of members of various racial and ethnic subgroups of women and men. Little attention has been paid to ethnic or racial differences in clinical research or to the relationship of these factors to socioeconomic status or sex. The 1994 IOM report also discusses trying to sort out the conceptualization of race, ethnicity, and socioeconomic status but still leaves investigators with a complex set of issues. Is race best defined by using genetic characteristics? Is it a valid category? Do genes determine race or is race a "societally constructed taxonomy that reflects the intersection of biological, cultural, socioeconomic, political and legal factors, as well as racism"(Williams et al., 1994)? Can race and ethnicity be usefully defined by using groups such as Hispanics, Asians and Pacific Islanders, American Indians and Alaskan Natives, African Americans, and whites? Do all Hispanics belong to one group or must they be divided into subgroups? How does one factor into research the values and desires of the community to be studied? Most crucial of all, how does the researcher deal with a legacy of mistrust about research held by many of these communities and fulfill the desires of each community to set its own research agenda?

To recruit and retain women and minorities as participants in clinical trials, some differences in the way trials are conducted may be necessary to accommodate the responsibilities of women in the remainder of their lives. However this is accomplished, we have left behind the assumption that adult males are the norm for people.

LENS 5: WOMEN OF CHILDBEARING AGE AND PREGNANT WOMEN ARE VULNERABLE AND NEED PROTECTION

For new biotechnology to be productively applied to women's health care issues, we need to be able to test new products in women of all ages. The 1994 IOM report recommends that investigators and institutional review boards not exclude people of reproductive age from participation in clinical studies. In the case of women of reproductive age, the potential for women to become pregnant during the study may not be used as a justification for precluding or limiting participation.

The same principle of inclusion is suggested in the report for pregnant women. Why should pregnant women be classified as vulnerable subjects in need of protection? Is society confusing the woman, who is an autonomous human being able to make decisions about herself (i.e., give a valid informed consent), with the fetus who may be vulnerable? If the fetus is vulnerable, who is a more appropriate person to make decisions about the future child than the one who will bear, love, and care for that child? With the inclusion of women in clinical trials, including women of childbearing age, we are moving away from protectionism. Women realize that there are advantages as well as burdens to their being included in clinical trials.

However, we need only to trace the history of research on human subjects to understand why we have protections built into the system. After the atrocities committed in the name of science on prisoners of war and civilians during World War II, a set of standards, called the Nuremberg Code, was drafted for judging the physicians and scientists who conducted these war-time human experiments (Reiser et al., 1989). The Nuremberg Code, developed in 1948, left the responsibility for action to the physicians and scientists involved in the research. The Nuremberg Code stimulated the development of other codes for protecting human subjects, for example, the Helsinki Declaration, which suggested review by others but again left the final responsibility in the hands of the physicians and scientists (World Medical Association, 1975).

Despite the development of such codes to provide guidance to health care professionals, flagrant abuses concerning the use of humans as research subjects continued to occur in the United States. In 1966, even though proper informed consent was not obtained, debilitated elderly patients at the Jewish Chronic Disease Hospital in Brooklyn were injected with live cancer cells to determine if the cells would be rejected (Faden and Beauchamp, 1986; Katz, 1972; Rothman, 1991). At about the same time, institutionalized children at Willowbrook were given hepatitis and watched to describe the natural history of the disease (Faden and Beauchamp, 1986; Katz, 1972; Rothman, 1991). Also in 1966, a series of 22 studies in which there were serious problems related to the use of vulnerable human subjects in unethical research experiments was exposed by Henry K. Beecher (1966) in a landmark speech.

In 1966 the U.S. Surgeon General first required all medical institutions that were funded by the Public Health Service (PHS) to have committees for reviewing human research protocols that were made up of scientists, clinicians, ethicists, and member of the community. In 1972 it was revealed that the Tuskegee Syphilis Study, begun in the 1930s, was still ongoing, which clearly demonstrated that the safety of research subjects was not protected in our country (Tuskegee Syphilis Study Ad Hoc Advisory Panel, 1973). Hearings held by the Senate Committee on Labor and Public Welfare in 1973 covered topics such as sterilization of mentally retarded people, research on human fetuses, and the use of prisoners in research.

Partially in response to these disclosures, the National Research Act of 1974 (P.L. 93-348) established the institutional review board as a refinement of the independent review committees that were already meeting. Congress also established the National Commission for Protection of Human Subjects of Biomedical and Behavioral Research to provide principles and guidelines for the use of human as subjects in clinical research. The commission identified three comprehensive ethical principles as an analytical framework to assist physicians and scientists, human subjects, and reviewers of research proposals in understanding the ethical issues inherent in such research (National Commission for Protection of Human Subjects of Biomedical and Behavioral Research, 1978). These principles were respect for persons, beneficence, and justice. Although the meanings of these terms are interpreted slightly differently today, these three principles remain the bedrock for human subject use.

A second stream of problems led to the protectionist environment that exists today with respect to women of childbearing age. Thalidomide, a drug used as a sleeping pill or for nausea of pregnancy, was approved in 20 countries, not including the United States. However, doctors began to note thousands of severe limb malformations caused by the drug, mainly in Eastern Europe.

Diethylstilbestrol was widely prescribed in the 1940s and 1950s to prevent miscarriage, despite a clinical trial that showed it to be ineffective. Twenty years later, the daughters of these women began to be diagnosed with a rare adenocarcinoma of the vagina. Even though the diethylstilbestrol was given as part of medical practice and not in drug trials, both of these events further encouraged the protectionist stance of excluding women of childbearing age and pregnant women from drug trials.

In 1975 the guidelines developed by the commission were incorporated into Department of Health and Human Services regulations stipulating the exclusion of pregnant women and fetuses from research except under certain limited circumstances. The protectionist stance became law. The tendency not to include women of childbearing age must be reversed and the section of the federal legislation classifying women as vulnerable needs to be reconsidered in light of the changing role of women and the burdens that must be borne if scientific research only addresses medication for adult males and postmenopausal women.

LENS 6: ONLY AGENTS OR DRUGS GIVEN TO THE MOTHER, NOT THE FATHER, CAN AFFECT THE EMBRYO OR FETUS

Another issue that is largely ignored by modern science relates to the role of male toxicity on the embryo or fetus when males are given drugs, because people generally assume that only substances given to women can have such an effect. This issue is well discussed in the 1994 IOM report.

Little research has been done on this topic and most of that has been done only in rats. Damage could occur via toxic substances acting on the DNA of developing sperm, because the progenitor cells are replicating their DNA and many remain in the testis. Also, postconception ejaculates may contain toxicants that can affect the embryo or fetus in utero (IOM, 1994). I have seen one exception to the general practice of assuming that males have no role in toxicity, and that was in a Proscar advertisement: "Proscar is generally well tolerated by men. However, women who are pregnant, or women who could become pregnant, should avoid the active ingredient in Proscar. If the active ingredient is absorbed by a woman who is pregnant with a male baby, it may cause the male baby to be born with abnormalities of the sex organs."

At present, scientists are doing little research in the area of male-mediated embryo effects. Men entering trials are not usually asked if they have pregnant wives or plan to have children soon, and methods are not generally mandated for contraception for men included in clinical trials. It is important for scientists to address the role of male-mediated toxicity to the fetus and to regard equitably the possible toxic effects from drugs or treatments given to both mother and father.

LENS 7: DRUG COMPANIES CAN AVOID LIABILITY BY EXCLUDING WOMEN OF CHILDBEARING AGE (AND PREGNANT WOMEN) FROM DRUG TRIALS

When companies maintain that they do not want to include women of childbearing age or pregnant women in clinical trials, the first reason they give is that they fear liability suits. The many factors relating to this topic are well discussed in the 1994 IOM report. Because legal action for research injury is most often based on negligence claims, the best protection from negligence suits is a valid informed consent process. Adult men and women can give valid informed consent for themselves. The fear is that there could be liability if there is injury to a future child, because it is uncertain whether either or both parents can give valid informed consent for that future child. Yet despite the fear, few cases were found in which a child injured in utero during a clinical trial later successfully sued the company. One likely reason for this is that pregnant women and women of childbearing age have generally been excluded from trials.

However, with the increase in scientific knowledge about differences between men and women, legal liability is changing. Pharmaceutical companies may be sued for adverse pregnancy outcomes resulting from including women in the trial who are or might become pregnant or they may be sued by women who have adverse outcomes from taking pharmaceuticals because women were excluded from the trials.

At present pregnant women are classed as vulnerable subjects (45 CFR 46 Subpart B) and are grouped with fetuses, prisoners, mentally disabled people, and children. They can only be included in trials in certain situations. The inclusion of pregnant women is a very difficult issue, and there are many barriers to their inclusion. For example, the background incidence of developmental problems is high, 20 to 30 percent of recognized pregnancies end in miscarriage, and 3 to 8 percent of babies have birth defects.

An IOM (1989) study of obstetrical malpractice showed that 50 percent of all malpractice awards come from obstetrical cases and that malpractice cases are generally jury cases. Even when there were few or no data showing that the physician had committed malpractice, juries tended to make awards to babies with serious developmental problems because of the human tragedy involved, the lack of other means to provide care, and the perception that insurance companies have a lot of money.

However, there are good reasons to have women, including women of childbearing age, participate in trials. The federal regulations on the inclusion of pregnant women in clinical trials need to be reexamined because pregnant women take medications that have not been tested in pregnant women; pregnancy can change drug pharmacokinetics (absorption, distribution, and plasma volume); there would be closer scrutiny and presumably less fetal harm if women were first studied in clinical trials; and there are new understandings of the meaning of autonomy, benefits and harms, and justice with respect to women and their inclusion in trials.

What issues should be considered regarding possible changes in the federal regulations for pregnant women? In which phases of clinical trials might pregnant women be considered? Should pregnant women ever be included before teratogenicity results are known? How important is a drug for pregnant women? Have drugs first been tested in nonpregnant women? What stage of pregnancy is involved? Are there other methods for determining adverse effects of the drug in pregnancy? What are the liability issues? If testing of drugs in pregnant women is deemed necessary, a system of reimbursement for injuries caused by the research might be one way to handle the liability issue.

LENS 8: CONGRESS HAS OBJECTIVE CRITERIA AND MECHANISMS TO DETERMINE HOW AND WHERE MONEY SHOULD BE SPENT

Congress needs a better way to determine how much to spend on various areas of disease research, including the evaluation of morbidity, mortality, quality of life, and scientific opportunity, instead of being so affected by special-interest groups. Special-interest groups can and are influencing Congress to advance their own policy positions with respect to clinical research. Pressure from women's groups was a major factor in the passage of the NIH Revitalization Act related to women in clinical trials and in the $210 million awarded to the Department of Defense funding for breast cancer research.

How the lack of research on women's health compromised the health information on women was documented by the 1985 PHS Task Force on Women's Health, which led to a new NIH policy in 1986 to encourage researchers to include women in clinical research. In 1990 public attention was again focused on the lack of women in clinical research; a General Accounting Office (GAO) report evaluating the 1986 NIH policy noted that there were few recorded data on inclusion and that many large NIH studies included only men. In September 1990 William Raub created the Office of Research on Women's Health. In 1991 NIH and the Alcohol, Drug Abuse and Mental Health Administration instructed grant applicants to include women and racial and ethnic groups in clinical study populations unless clear and compelling reasons are given for their exclusion.

In 1992 a second GAO report on inclusion of women in clinical trials reported that "for more than 60 percent of the drugs, the representation of women in the test population was less than the representation of women in the population with the corresponding disease." In addition, drug companies often did not analyze differences in trial data due to sex despite a Food and Drug Administration (FDA) guideline that encouraged such analysis.

The federal agencies that should be providing leadership on these issues, FDA and NIH, seem to have been as confused as the rest of us. Had they reacted more effectively and sooner, we might be in a better position now. For example, women of childbearing age have been omitted from the early phases of drug trials (except in life-threatening conditions), as recommended by the 1977 FDA guidelines. These remained in place until July 22, 1993, when FDA published for public comment new guidelines that modify and revise the earlier version. The new guidelines suggest that subjects in a clinical study should reflect the population that will receive the drug when it is marketed. The new guidelines encourage, but do not require, that women be included in the early phases of drug trials. They suggest that women and men be included in the same trial to permit direct comparison by sex within the study and that there be pharmacokinetic studies of variations with regard to menstrual cycles, pre- and postmenopausal effects of estrogen replacement therapy, and contraceptives. The guidelines use the informed consent process to advise women about fetal risk but they remain silent on recommendations for pregnant women.

LENS 9: CONGRESS HAS GOOD ADVICE AND MECHANISMS TO DESIGN RESEARCH STUDIES TO MEET THESE GOALS.

The 1993 NIH Revitalization Act states, "In conducting or supporting clinical research . . . the Director of NIH shall . . . ensure that: Women are included as subjects in each project of such research; and members of minority groups are included as subjects of such research." Regarding the design of clinical trials it states, "The Director of NIH shall ensure that the trial is designed and carried out in a manner sufficient to provide for a valid analysis of whether the variables being studied in the trial affect women or members of minority groups, as the case may be, differently than other subjects in the trial."

The law requires a valid subgroup analysis for women and men and members of minority groups but does not state how to subclassify minorities. To have statistical significance, each trial would be very large and expensive. Although I agree with the intent of Congress to gain inclusion for women and minorities in clinical trials, this legislation has created a difficult situation for investigators applying for NIH support of clinical trials. The 1994 IOM report suggests that the problem of inclusion is better solved on the more general level of a research agenda, not on the basis of individual experiments.

SUMMARY

There are many technologies being developed that will need appropriate testing in both men and women. We must ensure that these technologies work before they become accepted medical practice. To do this, society must rapidly confront and solve the problem of including women in the research process, especially women of childbearing age and pregnant women. We must also confront, study, and resolve ethical, legal, social, and economic issues related to the use of these technologies before they are introduced into clinical practice.

REFERENCES

Beecher, H. L. 1966. Ethics and clinical research. N. Engl. J. Med. 274:1354-1360.

Black, W. C., and H. G. Welch. 1993. Advances in diagnostic imaging and overestimations of disease prevalence and the benefits of therapy. N. Engl. J. Med. 328:1237-1243.

Crossan, J. D. 1988, The Dark Interval. Towards a Theology of Story. Sonoma, Calif.: Polebridge Press.

Faden, R. R., and T. L. Beauchamp. 1986. A History and Theory of Informed Consent. New York: Oxford University Press.

Food and Drug Administration. 1977. General Consideration for the Clinical Evaluation of Drugs. Rockville, Md.: FDA.

Food and Drug Administration. 1993. Guidelines for the Study and Evaluation of Gender Differences in the Clinical Evaluation of Drugs; Notice. Fed. Regist. 58:39406-39416.

General Accounting Office. 1990. Summary of Testimony Given by Mark. V. Nadel on Problems in Implementing the NIH Policy on Women in Study Populations. Washington, D.C.: GAO.

General Accounting Office. 1992. Women's Health: FDA Needs to Ensure More Study of Gender Difference in Prescription Drug Testing. GAO/HRD-93-17. Washington, D.C.: GAO.

Hellinger, F. J. 1993. The use of health services by women with HIV infection. Health Serv. Res. 28: 543-561.

Institute of Medicine. 1989. Medical Professional Liability and the Delivery of Obstetrical Care. Vol. 1. Washington, D.C.: National Academy Press.

Institute of Medicine. 1994. Women and Health Research. Ethical and Legal Issues of Including Women in Clinical Studies. Vol. 1. A. C. Mastroianni, R. Faden, and D. Federman, eds. Washington, D.C.: National Academy Press,

Khan, S. S., S. Nessim, R. Gray, L. S. Czer, A. Chaus, and J. Matloff. 1990. Increased mortality of women in coronary artery bypass surgery: evidence for referral bias. Ann. Intern. Med. 112:561-567.

Katz, J. 1972. Experimentation with Human Beings. New York: Russell Sage Foundation.

Kuhn, T. S. 1970. The Structure of Scientific Revolutions. 2nd ed. Chicago: University of Chicago Press.

Lurie, N., J. Slater, P. McGovern, J. Eskstrum, L. Quam, and K. Margokis. 1993. Preventive care for women. Does the sex of the physician matter? N. Engl. J. Med. 329:478-482.

Miller, J. B. 1989. The emerging post modern world. Pp. 1-19 in Postmodern Theology Christian Faith in a Pluralistic World, F. B. Burnham, ed. San Francisco: Harper.

Minkoff, H. L., and J. A. DeHovitz. 1991. Care of women infected with the human immunodeficiency virus. JAMA 266:2253-2258.

Multiple Risk-Factor Intervention Trial Group. 1977. Statistical design considerations in the NHLI multiple risk factor intervention trial (MRFIT). J. Chronic Dis. 30:261-275.

National Commission for the Protection of Human Subjects of Biomedical and Behavioral Research. 1978. The Belmont Report: Ethical Principles and Guidelines for the Protection of Human Subjects of Research. Washington, D.C.: U.S. Government Printing Office.

Randall, T. 1993. Producers of videodisc programs strive to expand patient's role in medical decision-making process. JAMA 270:160-162.

Reiser, S. J., A. J. Dyke, and W. J. Curran, eds. 1989. Ethics in Medicine. Historical Perspectives and Contemporary Concerns. Cambridge, MA: Massachusetts Institute of Technology Press.

Rothman, D. J. 1991. Strangers at the Bedside: A History of How Law and Bioethics Transformed Medical Decisionmaking. New York: Basic Books.

Steering Committee of the Physician Health Study Research Group. 1989. Final report on the aspirin component of the ongoing physician 'health study.' N. Engl. J. Med 321:129-35.

Tobin, J. N., S. Wassertheil-Smoller, J. P. Wexler, R. M. Steingart, N. Budner, L. Lense, J. Wachspress. 1987. Sex bias in considering coronary bypass surgery. Ann. Intern. Med. 107:19-25.

Tuskegee Syphilis Study Ad Hoc Advisory Panel. 1973. Final Report. Washington, D.C.: Public Health Service.

Williams, D. R., R. Lanizzo-Maurey, and R. C. Warren. 1994. The concept of race and health status in America. Pub. Health Rep. 109:26-41.

World Medical Association. 1975. Guiding Medical Doctors in Biomedical Research Involving Human Subjects. Adopted by the 18th World Medical Assembly, Helsinki, Finland, 1964, revised in 1975.

Part 5

THE ROLE OF GOVERNMENT IN THE
DEVELOPMENT OF BIOTECHNOLOGY

S cientists, industrialists, and the general public all have different expectations of government. Today the role of government in the lives
of Americans is being widely questioned, with many people arguing forcefully that government has become too big and intrusive: that it is
time to roll back excessive government regulation and reassert market
forces. This ongoing public debate serves as a backdrop to the final section of this book, which examines the role governments have played (and
continue to play) in the development of biotechnology not only in the
United States but also in other major industrialized countries.

In Chapter 19, Louis Lasagna of Tufts University School of Medicine
compares and contrasts drug approval policies in the United States, Europe, and Japan. He notes that although most biopharmaceutical products originate in the United States and begin clinical trials here, they are
usually marketed first in Europe. As a result of the longer time required
for clinical studies in the United States, together with lengthy and stringent product review processes, fewer new drugs are introduced in this
country than anywhere else except Norway. By contrast, Lasagna points
out, other industrialized countries regulate drug prices and pharmaceutical industry profits much more strictly than does the United States.

The former associate director for science in the Clinton White House,
M. R. C. Greenwood, is in no doubt that the U.S. government has played
a crucial role in nurturing research on biotechnology and will continue to
play an important role in supporting the growth of the burgeoning biotechnology industry. In Chapter 20, Greenwood asserts that federal fund-

223

ing of basic research was critical to the development of biotechnology and that the government's role now is to promote policies that help the biotechnology industry grow. The Clinton administration's efforts in this regard, according to Greenwood, include promoting partnerships between federal laboratories and the private sector and authorizing tax incentives to stimulate investment in biotechnology companies.

The final chapter in this section provides an insight into the U.S. government's regulatory process. Although author Suzanne Giannini Spohn of the Environmental Protection Agency (EPA) focuses on the development of regulations by EPA, the general principles that she outlines are probably common to all government rule-making agencies. Noting that the regulatory process involves trying to resolve many conflicting interests, Giannini Spohn predicts that until a more solid knowledge base exists upon which to base risk assessment of biotechnology products and until these products gain wider public acceptance, the EPA's approach to their regulation likely will remain relatively conservative.

19

Comparison of U.S., European, and Japanese Policies Affecting Pharmaceutical and Biotechnology Development

LOUIS LASAGNA

Biotechnology-derived pharmaceutical products in the United States are regulated by our Food and Drug Administration (FDA), whose philosophy has been that the processes by which new health care products are produced are in principle irrelevant to the scrutiny they undergo to gain approval for marketing. The decision as to whether a biotechnology drug will travel the regulatory pathway as a biologic (and hence under the jurisdiction of the Center for Biologics Evaluation Research [CBER]) or as a drug (and hence under the jurisdiction of the Center for Drug Evaluation Research [CDER]) is made case by case, although there is a 1991 working agreement between CBER and CDER that sets out general guidelines for the allocation of review authority. There are, however, implications of this decision, because a biologic requires a product license application instead of a new drug application, and every product license application must be accompanied by an establishment license application for the site of manufacture (Hawkins, 1990).

WORLDWIDE BIOPHARMACEUTICAL DEVELOPMENT

The patterns of worldwide development of biopharmaceuticals are of considerable interest (Bienz-Tadmor, 1993). In the decade ending in 1992, 14 different such products had been marketed in at least one country. If one counts identical versions of the original products, there was a total of 40 such products, 36 of them marketed in the United States, Europe, or Japan. Of the 14 new biological entities, 11 had been introduced in the

225

United States, all 14 somewhere in Europe (primarily in Germany, France, Italy, the United Kingdom, and Spain), and 10 in Japan.

A different picture emerges if one looks at all 40 products. Only 15 were on the market in the United States whereas 27 were available in Europe and 23 in Japan (2 of which were later removed from the market).

Although most biopharmaceuticals originated and began clinical trials in the United States, they tended to be marketed first in Europe. Why? Although regulatory review time was on average longer in the United States than in the average European country, it was about the same in Japan. More important, it would seem, was the time required for the clinical studies: just over 3 years in the United States (similar to Japan) but only 2 years in Europe. (Japan also suffered from a later entry into this market, with clinical testing having started about 2 years after the United States.)

In the major European countries and in Japan, many different companies have been able to market their products, even when their products are similar to one another, whereas in the United States generally only one version of each product is available. A partial explanation for many of these products lies in the provisions of the U.S. Orphan Drug Act, which prevents subsequent similar versions for the same indication from entering the market for 7 years.

U.S. LAG IN DRUG INTRODUCTION

In a way, biotechnology products in the decade in question conjure up the vision of the drug lag first documented in the 1970s by Wardell (1973, 1978). Wardell pointed out that drugs were introduced later in the United States than in the United Kingdom and that some of these drugs were important therapeutic advances. More recently, Andersson (1992) noted that the longest delays in the introduction of new drugs occur in the United States, Sweden, and Norway whereas shortest delays are generally found in the United Kingdom and (West) Germany. Regarding the introduction of new drugs, he noted that the United States and Norway have introduced far fewer than have any other industrialized countries.

One can only hope that the situation will not deteriorate further, because both FDA Commissioner Kessler and the Pharmaceutical Manufacturers Association have expressed concern about the growing backlog of biotechnology applications. In September 1992, Kessler said that he was worried about the biotechnology product pipeline; although drugs take an average of 20 months for approval, biologics average 40 months (PMA, 1992). According to Kessler, 3,000 biotechnology products entered the investigation stage in 1991, but only 6 to 12 are approved annually, and these products had been in the investigation pipeline for approximately 5 years. However, a major reorganization of CBER in January 1993, a new review scheme, 124 new staff additions, and a "refusal-to-file" policy may improve the situation.

BIOTECHNOLOGY PRODUCT DEVELOPMENT

It is not clear what effect the current movement toward international harmonization of regulatory requirements will have on biotechnology product development. European harmonization moves have been ongoing for some time, in observance of the 1992 deadline established by the Treaty of Rome in 1957, but it is problematic how much facilitation of drug registration has been achieved in the European Community (Donnely, 1993; Orzack et al., 1992). According to Orzack et al.:

> The abilities of national governments to protect public health seem threatened; health ministries and regulatory bodies may lose the prerogative of direct control of the domestic market for drugs approved in other countries or by a multinational agency; regulatory systems intended to monitor how well medicines meet international standards of safety, efficacy, and quality are seen as protectionist bodies, restricting trade among nations and as barriers to European unity.
>
> . . . The Community will in all likelihood try to resolve many of these problems. But the extent to which it can come up with workable and effective arrangements for pharmaceutical medicines is not clear. Will the proposed legislation speed evaluations? Can it aid the introduction of pharmaceuticals? If the EC [European Community] is to achieve a single market, its member states must support it and show the political will to cooperate. The EC may in time achieve its objective of a unified economic region within which goods (including pharmaceutical medicines), services, people, and capital may circulate without confronting restrictive national barriers, but when and how appear uncertain.

In the last few years, however, Europe, the United States, and Japan seem to have made substantial progress, at least in agreeing on certain kinds of technical requirements, including general toxicity testing, reproductive toxicology, clinical safety, good clinical practices, and dose-response trial designs, among others. Some of the trends support the hope that applications for product registration can profit not only by the elimination of needlessly extensive and prolonged animal toxicity testing, but from the possibility that different countries will accept the same filing format.

On November 19, 1993, a new regulation went into effect permitting FDA to share confidential commercial information with foreign regulatory bodies (but not the public) without the consent of the sponsor. Nevertheless, one has the feeling that we are a long way from an "international FDA" whose judgment would be binding on all developed countries, despite what seem to be moves in that direction. The European Committee for Proprietary Medicinal Products, for example, was supposed to facilitate the free movement of medicinal products, but its efficacy has been questionable, to say the least. It is almost impossible to imagine our FDA yielding approval authority to an international regulatory agency, given our history and politics. (A "super FDA" was dealt a cruel blow when the leading candidate for Drug Czar, Dr. Duilio Poggiolini, was put in prison in Italy for unsavory regulatory practices.)

DRUG PRICING AND REIMBURSEMENT

Market approval is, worldwide, infinitely less important than drug pricing and reimbursement. Every developed country except the United States has a formal governmental procedure for controlling pharmaceutical costs, and even the United States is moving rapidly away from a truly free market environment. The schemes used to this end are almost as numerous as the countries that have adopted them. It is far from clear whether each system is right even for the country adopting it, let alone desirable for other countries. Needless to say, research cannot thrive without investment of resources, and the biotechnology industry is particularly vulnerable to cost containment. Except for programs supported heavily by traditional pharmaceutical companies, small biotechnology firms are crucially dependent on venture capital to keep their research going until a product reaches the market. When that happy event occurs, there is the not-surprising desire to recoup past investment, reward investors, and plow more money into new research. Decisions about manufacturing are difficult as well. A new production plant may cost $25 million and the timing of its construction is tricky, given the uncertainties of FDA approval and the timing of the signal for ground-breaking.

Europe

Let us first consider Europe. As Heinz Redwood (In press) has put it, there are three principles in European public policy: solidarity (the conviction that society must provide health care to all), subsidiarity ("Eurocrats Keep Out whenever our own national bureaucrats can do the job at least as well"), and pharmapolitics, with its four strands (financial, medical, industrial, and electoral).

In all member states except Portugal, public drug spending has risen more rapidly than the national rate of inflation, and price controls have seemed to provide no modulating influence. The French have tried superimposing volume control over price control and are discussing sanctions for excessive prescribing by physicians. The British provide budgets for large medical practices, with financial incentives for underspending. Germany tried reference pricing without success but discovered a system that reduces drug prescribing. If the German national drug budget is overspent, the doctors' associations are responsible for the first 280 million DM (about $175 million) and the pharmaceutical industry is responsible for the next 280 million DM. The scheme has been in effect since January 1993 and is working even though 280 million DM is said to be only 1 percent of the German medical profession's income from treating patients under the government health system. (No one is tracking the effect of these prescribing cutbacks on the quality of health care.) Expenditures for drugs were 26.2 billion DM in 1992, the budget target for 1993 was 23.8 billion, and actual expenditures were 21.2 billion DM.

Only the United Kingdom has approached drug pricing with an imaginative scheme for keeping firms profitable but not excessively so. British politicians like the drug industry and are grateful for its products and for its positive contributions to the balance of trade. This British mechanism, called the Pharmaceutical Price Regulation Scheme (PPRS), is based on profits and operates at the level of a company's total business with the National Health Service, not individual products, the prices of which are set by each company. The basis is to be a return on capital used or, for some foreign firms, the return on sales. A target profit is set within an allowable range of 17 to 21 percent, with a 25 percent margin for error. Costs associated with sales are assessed on production expenses, distribution, information, research and development, general and administrative expenses, and promotion. The latter is limited to about 9 percent of sales, a lot less than is spent in other countries. Research and development averages around 20 percent of sales, substantially above the 14 percent that is typical of the rest of the developed world. In August 1993 the PPRS was renegotiated and renewed for 5 years. The terms will reduce profits by imposing an across-the-board reduction of 2.5 percent for 3 years, which began October 1, 1993. The U.K. approach is not without its critics, but it may be superior to other European approaches.

Japan

Japan is also unique. The Ministry of Health and Welfare sets a fee schedule for drugs. Physicians in Japan not only prescribe drugs, they also dispense them, and much of their income comes from the margin between drug acquisition prices and the fee schedule. Manufacturers need the loyalty of doctors, so they compete by maximizing this margin. Drug prices start high but come down rapidly in succeeding years, creating an incentive for doctors to prescribe newly marketed drugs. To contain drug costs, the government decreed eight price cuts for drugs in the period from 1981 to1992, with the squeeze being largely absorbed by the drug industry.

For this and other reasons, the Japanese industry is moving into the other two huge pharmaceutical markets: Europe and the United States. Japan, although a huge market by itself, cannot suffice to serve the income needs of an industry that wishes not just to survive, but to thrive. Biotechnology represents a part of that international effort.

For those who believe that Japanese scientists are only imitators, not innovators, the paper by Hawkins and Reich (1992) is necessary reading. They examined Japanese-originated ethical pharmaceuticals introduced in the United States during the past 30 years, looking for evidence of true innovation. They used the following requirements: structural novelty, biologic novelty, therapeutic importance, and economic success. They found that Japan not only had produced innovative compounds, but was responsible for some of the best-selling drugs in the U.S. market.

Japan also illustrates other interesting differences. It spends more than any other nation on pharmaceuticals (almost twice as much as the United States in 1990 and three times as much as the United Kingdom). Hence 30 percent of national health expenditure goes for medicines. Hospital stays are unbelievably long, mental health services are inadequate, and elderly people have one of the highest suicide rates in the world (Imamura, 1993).

Japan has almost no U.S.-style small biotechnology companies. Instead, such research is focused in large, well-established pharmaceutical, fermentation, or chemical companies. The Japanese government began stimulating interest in industrial biotechnology in the late 1970s and early 1980s. Many of the preferential treatment areas for federal grants are in biotechnology. By contrast, venture capital investors have been slow to show interest. However, large Japanese companies—pharmaceutical, chemical, and food—are becoming major investors in the U.S. biotechnology industry (National Research Council, 1992).

PATENT PROTECTION

In most countries, patent protection runs from the date of filing of the patent application. In the United States, patents date from the granting of the patent. In Japan, the patent term commences from the date of publication of the specification. Since the European Patent Convention of 1977, most European countries allow patent exclusivity for 20 years. In the United States, patent protection theoretically lasts for 17 years, but for pharmaceuticals the lengthy development and approval process (which usually occurs while the patent clock is ticking) in essence halves this amount. The 1984 Drug Price Competition and Patent Term Restoration Act provides for up to five years of increase in patent protection in certain cases. The terms of the General Agreement on Tariffs and Trade (GATT) and the North American Free Trade Agreement (NAFTA) provide for a patent term of 20 years from date of filing as well as for product and process patents for almost all types of inventions, including pharmaceuticals. Signatories are under a general obligation to comply with the agreement terms through implementing legislation.

In the 1960s and 1970s Japan was mainly licensing drugs from foreign countries and patent protection only applied to chemical processes. In 1976 a product patent system with 15 years of exclusivity was introduced. In 1980, responding to the problem of lengthy development times, Japan revised the law to ensure a minimum 6 years of exclusivity. In 1987 a further amendment provided for patent term restoration to a maximum of 5 years (Centre for Medicines Research, 1989).

THE FUTURE FOR BIOTECHNOLOGY

Will the United States maintain its strong biotechnology leadership in the future? Should our government be increasing financial incentives to encourage innovation, venture capital investment, and long-term strategic planning? The next century will be an interesting period in the history of global technology.

REFERENCES

Andersson, F. 1992. The drug lag issue: the debate seen from an international perspective. Int. J. Health Sci. 22:53-72.

Bienz-Tadmor, B. 1993. Biopharmaceuticals go to market: patterns of worldwide development. Biotechnology 11:168-172.

Centre for Medicines Research. 1989. Pharmaceutical Patents. The Stimulus to Medicines Research. Carshalton, Surrey, U. K.: CMR.

Donnely, M. 1993. Experience with the multi-state procedure: transition to the decentralized procedure. Drug Inf. J. 27:43-49.

Hawkins, E. S. 1990. Biotechnology in the United States pharmaceutical industry. Pharmaceut. Med. 4:229-302.

Hawkins, E. S., and M. R. Reich. 1992. Japanese-originated pharmaceutical products in the United States from 1960 to 1989: an assessment of innovation. Clin. Pharmacol. Ther. 51:1-11.

Imamura, K. 1993. A critical look at health research in Japan. Lancet 342:279-282.

National Research Council. 1992. U.S.–Japan Technology Linkages in Biotechnology. Challenges for the 1990s. Washington, D.C.: National Academy Press.

Orzack, L. H., K. I. Kaitin, and L. Lasagna. 1992. Pharmaceutical regulation in the European Community: barriers to single market integration. J. Health Polit. Policy Law 17:847-868.

PMA. 1992. PMA Newslett. Sept. 28: 4.

Redwood, H. 1994. Public policy trends in drug pricing and reimbursement in the European Community. International Symposium on Pricing and Reimbursement of Pharmaceuticals: An Evaluation of Cost-Containment Strategies, July 21-22, 1993. PharmacoEconomics 6(Suppl. 1):3-10.

Wardell, W. M. 1973. Introduction of new therapeutic drugs in the United States and Great Britain: an international comparison. Clin. Pharmacol. Ther. 14:773-790.

Wardell, W. M. 1978. The drug lag revisited: comparison by therapeutic area of patterns of drugs marketed in the United States and Great Britain from 1972 through 1976. Clin. Pharmacol. Ther. 24:499-524.

20

Expanding the Horizons of Biotechnology in the Twenty-first Century

M. R. C. GREENWOOD and RACHEL E. LEVINSON

The Clinton administration has embarked on an important initiative. Shortly after taking office, President Clinton and Vice President Gore released a report entitled "Technology for America's Economic Growth, A New Direction to Build Economic Strength." (Clinton and Gore, 1993). This document presents three key goals: 1) long-term economic growth that creates jobs and protects the environment, 2) a government that is more productive and more responsive to the needs of its citizens, and 3) world leadership in basic science, mathematics, and engineering.

The report outlined policies and initiatives that support efforts to attain the first goal. Vice President Gore's national performance review addressed the second goal. After becoming associated with the Office of Science and Technology Policy (OSTP), we began thinking about ways in which we might address the third goal. With the wonderful assistance of Drs. Neal Lane and Harold Varmus (directors of the National Science Foundation [NSF] and the National Institutes of Health [NIH], respectively), we have begun to develop a companion document to the technology policy report, one that will enunciate a presidential science policy for the twenty-first century, define a vision of science in the national interest, and describe the steps toward making this vision a reality.

As a first step toward achieving this goal, the OSTP in conjunction with the National Academy of Sciences convened a national forum entitled *Science in the National Interest: World Leadership in Basic Science, Mathematics, and Engineering*. The forum was held at the academy on January

31 and February 1, 1994, to identify opportunities and challenges facing our nation and to define the points of convergence between science policy and public policy. Fifteen organizations, including NSF; NIH; U.S. Department of Agriculture; Department of Energy (DOE); Department of Defense; American Association for the Advancement of Science; Carnegie Commission on Science, Technology, and Government; Industrial Research Institute; Dana Foundation; National Association of State Universities and Land Grant Colleges; and Association of American Universities cosponsored the forum, indicating its broad spectrum of interest and involvement across government, academia, and industry (Mervis, 1993).

Some of the key speakers at the forum included OSTP Director John Gibbons, Senator Barbara Mikulski, Senator Jay Rockefeller, Senator Tom Harkin, Representative George Brown, National Academy of Sciences President Bruce Alberts, and, of course, Neal Lane and Harold Varmus. Vice President Al Gore also attended and stressed his commitment to science, especially fundamental science. He emphasized the importance of the forum as critical to the process of developing a national science policy that will guide federal investment in the scientific enterprise. The following quote from Vice President Gore's speech captures and conveys the strongest elements of this administration's commitment to basic scientific research:

> It is clear to this Administration that the needs of scientists who are addressing basic questions about the nature of matter, the nature of our earth, the nature of the universe, the structure of thought, the biochemical structure of genetic inheritance, the interaction of environment and biological development, the modification of behavior and the design of social institutions, must be met. For their discoveries today will be the rich soil that will support the growth of innovations and applications that we can not yet foresee in the 21st Century. We are keenly aware that the Federal investment in funding their research and supporting their laboratories and their education is an investment in our Nation's future. The challenge we face is how to make this investment with the limited resources we have available today.

There is much to be proud of in U.S. science. Our nation is without peer in many areas of scientific outcomes, whether we measure that success by the award of Nobel prizes, the type and number of discoveries and publications, or the potential for a new industrial, informational revolution. Clearly, we are privileged to be in a time of extraordinary opportunity and excitement. However, the sad truth is that we are also facing the reality of unprecedented fiscal constraints that force some very difficult choices in allocating the federal budget.

RESEARCH AND DEVELOPMENT IN FY 1995

President's Budget Request

On February 7, 1994, the president transmitted to Congress his budget request for fiscal year (FY)1995 (Table 20-1). The proposed budget recognizes research and development (R&D) funding as a priority investment. Within an overall freeze on discretionary spending that forced cuts in hundreds of programs, the president proposed an increase of 4 percent for R&D spending relative to what we are spending now as a necessary investment in the future. This comes to a total of over $71 billion ($73 billion with facilities), up $2.5 billion over 1994. Within this table, you may be particularly interested to note that the president has proposed a 4.7 percent increase for NIH, a 10 percent increase for university-based research and education funded by NSF, and a 6 percent increase overall.

While maintaining our overall investment in R&D, we are also shifting our R&D spending to increase the focus on new relevant national goals. The president has proposed an increase for R&D investments in areas that are directly relevant to strengthening our economic security, improving our quality of life, and maintaining our national security in a changing international environment. To accomplish this, the budget pro-

TABLE 20-1 Maintain the Investment: Research & Development (R&D) from 1993 to 1995 (dollar amounts in millions)

R&D by Agency (w/o Facilities)	1993 Actual	1994 Enacted	1995 Proposed	Change from 1994 to 1995[a]
Defense	38,617	35,538	36,971	1,433[4]
Health and Human Services	10,336	11,033	11,484	451[4]
(National Institutes of Health)	(9,775)	(10,349)	(10,861)	(512[5])
Commerce	667	919	1,204	284[31]
National Science Foundation	1,882	2,026	2,220	194[10]
National Aeronautics and Space Administration	8,090	8,493	8,597	105[1]
Transportation	578	617	692	75[12]
Environmental Protection Agency	508	536	582	46[9]
Agriculture	1,335	1,393	1,394	1[0]
Energy	5,827	6,054	6,052	(2[-0])
Other	1,910	1,876	1,833	(43[-2])
Total R&D	69,750	68,484	71,029	2,545[4]

[a]Percent change given in brackets.

posal includes R&D increases in such areas as biomedical research, our national information infrastructure, manufacturing technologies, environmental technologies, transportation, and dual-use technologies.

Throughout the R&D budget we propose to continue to expand partnerships with the private sector. This is the single best way to leverage our science and technology investments to ensure that those investments are relevant to the real-world problems and challenges facing our industries, state and local governments, etc. The budget includes increases in funding, for example, for cooperative research efforts and technology transfer programs (including manufacturing technology extension centers) that may be expected to have a positive effect on advances in biotechnology.

We want to ensure continued leadership in fundamental science through continued investments in basic science, math, and engineering research. This fundamental research drives our basic understanding of our world and its problems and is the seedbed for the new technologies and new options of the future. It represents our most important investment over the long term in our security (broadly defined) and our quality of life.

Human Genome Project

One example of how designated investments have fared in the FY 1995 budget request is the Human Genome Project, a "big science" effort managed cooperatively under the aegis of NIH and the DOE Office of Energy Research (Table 20-2). For FY 1995, the president has proposed $241 million to fund the DOE and NIH genome efforts. This represents an increase of $42 million, or 21 percent over the 1994 budget. Even if the purse strings were loose, this would look good. There is good reason for such optimism about genome research in the White House.

Alexander Pope once wrote that "the proper study of Man is Man." For what is daily being revealed about us as a result of this revolutionary effort, the Human Genome Project could easily be the most important organized scientific effort in the history of mankind. This is an historic research effort that will analyze the structure of human DNA and determine the location and sequence of the estimated 100,000 human genes that constitute the human blueprint. As you heard earlier in this forum from Tom Caskey and others, accomplishment of this goal will allow the identification of the genetic basis of a wide array of diseases, profoundly change the practice of medicine, provide a powerful stimulus for the biotechnology industry, and radically alter the future of biomedical research.

The Human Genome Project may be thought of by many as a "big science" project, but it is quite different from other such projects. First,

TABLE 20-2 Human Genome Project Budget (dollar amounts in millions)

	FY 1993 Actual	FY 1994 Current Estimate	FY 1995 President's Budget
National Institutes of Health	106.1	128.7	152.0
Department of Energy[a]	64.5	68.0	88.6
TOTAL	70.6	196.7	240.6

[a]Salaries and expenses of Department of Energy employees devoted to this effort are not included.

although it is centrally coordinated, it is being carried out by hundreds of investigators at dozens of research centers nationwide. Second, it has been producing beneficial results since it began and has already woven itself seamlessly into the fabric of biomedical research. Third, there is a strong and essential emphasis on creativity and innovation and a tight synthesis of science and technology. This has encouraged some of the best and brightest people in the country to invest their talents in achieving these ambitious goals.

NIH and DOE are the key agencies managing this project in the United States, but it is international in its scope and many other countries are making significant contributions, both scientifically and financially. The project has powerful implications for the future health and vigor of the American economy. Already new biotechnology companies are springing up across the country, ready to take advantage of the commercial opportunities generated by this project; 10 new companies were founded in the past year alone. These companies hope to capitalize on the advances in technology that have made it feasible to even consider sequencing the entire human genome.

The project evolved from decades of fundamental science research, involving many researchers from a broad spectrum of scientific disciplines, including disciplines beyond biology and medicine; it requires the skills and expertise of computer scientists, engineers, robotics experts, physicists, chemists, ethicists, lawyers, sociologists, and theologians. The project has also presented a complex challenge of information storage and access. The project illustrates the way in which fundamental science demands rapid access to large amounts of information. It might be said that the genome project is devoted to uncovering nature's information infrastructure. Powerful information superhighways are already being developed and used to allow researchers, physicians, companies, and the public to take full advantage of this remarkable treasure.

The project was finally initiated after several years of vigorous scientific debate about its merits. Today it is indisputable that the Human Genome Project is already providing researchers with powerful tools to rapidly and efficiently search for disease genes. The recent identification of a major gene for colon cancer illustrates these relationships very well: discovery of the gene will pave the way for a diagnostic test to identify individuals at high risk, which may include as many as 1 million Americans. This is particularly significant because careful medical surveillance and early detection vastly improves the outcome for individuals with this common inherited disease. A similar story is unfolding for breast cancer, with the identification of a major susceptibility gene expected in the near future.

A spectacular example of society's investment in basic biological research, and the way that research sometimes yields totally unexpected connections to problems important to human health and welfare, was described by Mark Peifer (1993). He discussed two articles appearing in the December 10 issue of *Science* that establish a link among human colon cancer, epithelial cell adhesion molecules, and pattern formation in the fruit fly *Drosophila*. Peifer makes the point that "the discovery of this unexpected protein-protein interaction is bound to stimulate much activity in three no longer disparate fields of research."

CROSS-DISCIPLINARY LINKAGES

One lesson we can learn from this example is that the likelihood of identifying such unexpected connections is greatly enhanced if we can speed the exchange of meaningful information among scientists, even those in apparently unrelated fields that may turn out to be related after all. This is an important concept that can be reasonably extended from the genome project to biotechnology and to science in its entirety.

Another lesson is that increasingly we must appreciate that the notion of unrelated fields is not particularly helpful and will prove meaningless in the twenty-first century. The pages of *Science* are replete with descriptions of squabbling within disciplines, such as the "biology-culture" gap within the field of anthropology. Yet we are increasingly impressed with the unifying links between disciplines and the value of identifying or establishing those links to advance what amounts to a multidisciplinary understanding of nature. Surely our ability to combat disease, solve our pressing social problems, and ensure our nation's future prosperity and security will grow out of a truly comprehensive understanding. The cross-disciplinary nature of the biotechnology toolbox illustrates this lesson rather graphically. How many of you were forced to master database searching methods to look for gene homologies or even to see what your competitors were up to? How many bioengineers went back to school to catch up on the latest in molecular biology?

What we are learning about the genetics of colon cancer and breast cancer suggests the likelihood that all of us carry at least some genetic predisposition to illness. The human genome project thus has clear consequences for health care, because it will provide individuals with the ability to determine their risks for future disease, allowing development of individualized programs of lifestyle alterations and medical surveillance designed to maintain wellness.

The identification of disease susceptibility that can be ameliorated by behavioral change brings up a crucial public health challenge that we will only be able to meet with the assistance of fundamental research in the social and behavioral sciences. We know that 5 of the10 leading causes of death are linked to behavior—the way we eat and the way we live—yet we know little about how to effect lasting positive behavioral change.

The economic benefit of helping large numbers of people adopt and sustain healthy behaviors and thereby avoid the medical costs of treating major chronic diseases such as heart disease, certain cancers, diabetes, hypertension, stroke, and osteoporosis is enormous. Because rising medical costs are the biggest contributor to our current inflationary spiral, the savings produced by positive behavioral change would substantially reduce the economic burden that medical costs represent to our society.

CHALLENGES BY AND FOR BIOTECHNOLOGY

The Human Genome Project provides a glimpse into the future of biomedical science. Biotechnology expands that vision and shows how the different disciplines can work synergistically, applying the tools and skills of physicists, bioengineers, and materials scientists to problems in bioprocessing; theoretical mathematicians, pharmacologists, and physicians to rational drug development; and, on a global scale, environmental ecologists, biochemists, and computer systems engineers to bioremediation and environmental restoration.

Biotechnology also challenges our current notions of integrated systems and feedback loops simply because of the rapid pace with which discoveries are put into practice and diffuse into many areas of application. Our traditional mechanisms for overseeing the support, application, and commercialization of new technologies have not been able to keep up with the explosion of growth in the biotechnology industries. This deficiency begins with the funding of technology development; some of our most important work that might advance an entire field has gone begging for resources because it falls between the cracks of programs offered by

NIH or NSF. This is particularly true, for example, for funding the development of new reagents and instruments.

It is painfully apparent that the public has not been adequately informed about the benign nature of biotechnology food products, for example, that pose absolutely no health risks but are still the target of antibiotechnology campaigns. Our regulatory systems are struggling valiantly to provide an appropriate, scientifically sound framework for product review and, at the same time, provide guidance to the applicants and the public to ensure a credible and rigorous oversight process.

As more biotechnology products attain commercial viability, intellectual property protection becomes more crucial on both the domestic and international fronts. This issue may seem tangential to the research concerns, but the absence of protection measures has an immediate and resounding effect on the ability to raise investment capital to fund biotechnology start-ups, which are already hampered somewhat by other uncertainties, such as public acceptance, regulatory approval, and a relatively long lead time between the lab and the marketplace.

Although the U.S. biotechnology industry is generally regarded as the world leader, no one is, or should be, complacent about our situation. There are signs indicating that biotechnology is at a particularly critical juncture right now, and the future vitality of our domestic capability may rest on what we in the administration and Congress and our partners in industry and academia can accomplish together in the coming several years. The Clinton administration has taken a very strong position that recognizes the critical role technology must play in stimulating and sustaining the long-term economic growth that creates high-quality jobs and protects our environment and the importance of biotechnology to our success in these areas.

The ability to enlist the cooperation of the forces of nature and put them to work in solving many of the problems we face today, such as feeding and providing energy to a growing population, improving human health, undoing some of the damage man has wrought on the global ecosystem, and sustaining our natural resources, resulted directly from government-funded basic research.

THE NATIONAL SCIENCE AND TECHNOLOGY COUNCIL AND THE BIOTECHNOLOGY RESEARCH SUBCOMMITTEE

Like other emerging industries, biotechnology is moving toward a phase in which much of the information necessary for advanced product and process development will be proprietary. However, this industry is one that will continue to look to the kind of fundamental scientific research that is supported through NIH, NSF, and other federal agencies.

For FY 1995, the administration is not conducting a comprehensive budget analysis of federal support for biotechnology research as was performed for the two previous years by the Biotechnology Research Subcommittee under the Federal Coordinating Council for Science, Engineering and Technology. Unfortunately, this has been interpreted to mean that we have phased out the activities of the Biotechnology Research Subcommittee. This is not so. On November 23, 1993, the president signed an executive order establishing the National Science and Technology Council (NSTC), which he will chair. The charge to this new cabinet-level council is to establish clear national goals for federal science and technology investments and to ensure that science and technology policies and programs are developed and implemented to contribute effectively to those national goals.

Private sector involvement with the NSTC will be essential to developing successful science and technology policies that will help American businesses achieve sustainable growth, create high-quality jobs, and maintain our academic and research institutions' world leadership in science, engineering, and mathematics. To ensure that federal science and technology policies reflect U.S. national needs, the president also established the President's Committee of Advisors on Science and Technology, which will advise the president on science and technology issues and assist the NSTC in securing private sector involvement in its activities. Committee members will be appointed by the president and will include distinguished individuals from industry, education, research institutions, nongovernmental organizations, and other sources.

As one of the first actions taken under this new policy coordination and implementation mechanism, we made certain that the efforts of the Biotechnology Research Subcommittee would continue under the new committee structure. This subcommittee will operate under the aegis of a single, overarching committee, the Committee on Fundamental Science, which is cochaired by Drs. Lane , Varmus, and Greenwood. The Biotechnology Research Subcommittee will continue to provide government-wide coordination and focus for biotechnology research in the various federal departments and agencies. Biotechnology will also receive attention in at least two other of the nine NSTC committees (e.g., Health, Safety, & Food; Environment and Natural Resources).

FEDERAL INVESTMENT IN BIOTECHNOLOGY

Under the NSTC, we will focus on extending the scientific and technical foundations necessary to the development of biotechnology, developing the human resources necessary to biotechnology, facilitating the transfer of biotechnology research discoveries to commercial applications, and

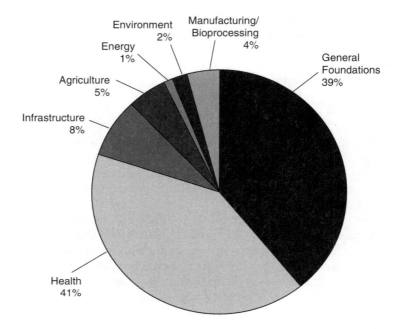

FY 1994: $4,299.3 M

FIGURE 20-1   Federal investment in biotechnology research by research area.

realizing the benefits of biotechnology for human health, agriculture, and the restoration and protection of the environment (Figure 20-1). The Biotechnology Research Subcommittee is developing strategic plans for federal research in agricultural, environmental, and marine and aquatic biotechnology and for manufacturing and bioprocessing technology.

Biotechnology research and development are supported through several other mechanisms. One of those is the Advanced Technology Program, administered by the Department of Commerce through the National Institute for Standards and Technology (NIST). The program is designed to promote the economic growth and competitiveness of U.S. business and industry by accelerating the development and commercialization of promising high-risk technologies with substantial potential for enhancing the nation's economy. The program's research priorities are set through an interactive process with industry, by means of competitive proposals from industry and academia for developing and commercializing innovative technologies. Out of 400 industry responses to a recent Advanced Technology Program announcement, 50 were in the biotechnology area. On January 12, 1994, NIST hosted a workshop on biotechnology to explain the procedures necessary to obtain support through the program and to solicit industry input on setting research priorities that meet the program selection criteria.

Instructions have been given to federal laboratories to devote more of their budgets to R&D partnerships with civilian industry. We are emphasizing increased use of cooperative, cost-shared research and development agreements (CRADAs) as well as other cooperative arrangements. One of the first CRADAs initiated by NIH is noteworthy in several respects. This agreement with Genetic Therapy Inc. capitalized on technology and expertise in the NIH laboratories of Drs. French Anderson, Michael Blaese, and Steven Rosenberg to launch a new company, a new form of treatment for genetic and other diseases, and a new industry sector, that is, gene therapy. Since the first human gene transfer trial initiated in 1988, NIH has approved more than 50 clinical gene therapy trials at centers across the nation. Studies involving revolutionary approaches to the treatment of cystic fibrosis, severe combined immune deficiency, advanced melanoma, and acquired immune deficiency syndrome are now underway or are about to begin. These represent tremendous health care and economic opportunities for this country.

Reflecting its growth dynamics, biotechnology depends heavily on the public and private investment markets to finance start-up and follow-on financing. Although we hear differing views on how long the window may remain open for biotechnology company public offerings, some are doing quite well right now. Biotechnology firms have generally been able to raise cash for the initial stages of operation, but second and third rounds of capital financing, which are necessary to bridge the gap between research and profit generation from marketable products, are more difficult to come by. A bottleneck is developing as start-up companies attempt to move forward into development, testing, and marketing: the expensive part of the process. As much as $5 billion to $10 billion may be needed just to develop the 100 biotechnology products currently in clinical trials.

The administration has taken some steps to improve the long-term, lower-cost availability of capital. The president has signed into law tax incentives for private-sector investment in R&D and new business formation, including a targeted reduction in the capital gains tax for investment in small businesses. We also continue to push on reducing federal deficits that siphon off savings that otherwise could flow to private capital markets.

The 1991 Office of Technology Assessment report on biotechnology in a global economy cited the research and experimentation tax credit as a key issue for congressional consideration in protecting U.S. industrial innovation and international competitiveness. In the past the effectiveness of this credit was seriously undermined because it was extended 1 year at a time. Under those conditions companies cannot accurately project the real costs of a given R&D project. R&D, by its nature, requires long-term investment, and businesses will be reluctant to make such commitments without a permanent research and experimentation tax credit. The tax credit was reauthorized for 3 years and we will continue to work toward our goal of making it permanent.

REGULATORY POLICY

We need a thoughtful, sensible, and, above all, clear regulatory framework that will encourage innovation and enable us to meet our national social objectives efficiently. As part of the technology initiative, the president and vice president stated that, "We can promote technology as a catalyst for economic growth by . . . directly supporting the development, commercialization and deployment of new technology" and "To improve the environment for private sector investment and create jobs, we will ensure that Federal regulatory policy encourages investment in innovation and technology development that achieve the purposes of the regulation at the lowest possible cost."

The Clinton administration welcomes open discussion and debate as key ingredients in developing successful regulations. Only through public dialogue can we develop regulations that address the necessary questions in a way that facilitates decision making by the government, increases certainty and predictability for industry at the lowest practical cost, and is demonstrably fair to the public interest.

It is the responsibility of the government to provide an effective and credible regulatory system. The biotechnology industry wants this as the best means to ensure public confidence in and acceptance of the products of biotechnology. There is no better antidote to the actions of anti-biotechnology activists than an informed public and an open debate.

CONCLUSION

Biotechnology offers great promise for the future and has the potential to affect nearly every facet of our lives. The keys to successful innovation and commercialization will be a strong basic research program, fiscal and economic tax policies that encourage investment, a rational regulatory policy, and an educated public. The Clinton administration will help sustain the strong research base for biotechnology and will offer a forum for biotechnology advocates and critics to reach consensus on how various biotechnology products can benefit our society.

This administration will work with the research communities in the public and private sectors and the American people to build that consensus, so that 10 years from now we can look back and say that the 1990s were the decade of continued vigorous research and of the successful commercialization of biotechnology and biotechnology products in the United States and throughout the world.

Biotechnology offers the science policy community at large a unique opportunity to forge linkages among the scientific disciplines and among the elements of the research community located in the government, in our institutions of higher education, and in the private sector. As policy-makers, we see our responsibility as one of fostering these nascent relationships and attempting to foresee and forestall the emergence of barriers to progress. We have the support of the president's science adviser and the administration in conveying their firm commitment to expanding the horizons of biotechnology and, indeed, for science more broadly, into the twenty-first century.

Paraphrasing Vice President Gore's recent remarks: We simply cannot afford to take the narrow view of science, looking only at immediate results. We have to cast our eyes ahead a few years, a few decades, a century or more, and imagine the unimaginable. There is much to do, but we have made a good start and have the will to continue.

REFERENCES

Clinton, W. J., and A. Gore. 1993. Technology for America's Ecomonic Growth, A New Direction to Build Economic Strength. Washington, D.C.: U.S. Government Printing Office.

Mervis, J. 1993. U. S. research forum fails to find a common front. Science 263:752. Office of Technology Assessment, B. Brown, ed. 1991. Biotechnology in a Global Economy. Washington, D.C.: U.S. Government Printing Office.

Peifer, M. 1993. Cancer, catenins, and cuticle pattern: a complex connection. Science 262:1667-1668.

21

The Making of Environmental Policy Decisions

SUZANNE GIANNINI SPOHN

S imply stated, the mission of the U.S. Environmental Protection Agency (EPA) is to protect human health and the environment. The potential environmental benefits that biotechnology products can provide are enormous: safer, less toxic pesticides; bioremediation agents to restore a degraded environment to its previous quality; more environment-friendly mining and oil-recovery processes, and pollution prevention in fossil fuel extraction and refining.

The ecological effect of large-scale, deliberate environmental releases of genetically engineered organisms is not simple to predict. This is especially true in the area of soil ecology and ecosystems processes, which are enormously complex and about which very little is understood. In the face of this kind of uncertainty, how does EPA decide what are acceptable levels of risk? In other words, how does EPA set regulatory policy?

To answer this question, I first need to make it clear that EPA is a regulatory agency, distinct from other federal agencies such as the National Science Foundation and the National Institutes of Health, whose primary mission is research. As a regulatory agency, EPA is an arm of the executive branch of the federal government, and our primary function is to implement the laws passed by the Congress that concern the environment.

Federal acts or laws are usually fairly broadly written directives from the Congress either requiring people or corporations to do something or prohibiting them from doing something else. These laws very rarely

This article represents the views of the author and it does not necessarily represent the official position of the U.S. Environmental Protection Agency.

specify in great detail how these actions are to be implemented. For example, what technology will be used to attain the desired results? Who is going to pay for or maintain the technology? How will violations be defined or detected? What kinds of evidence or data must be supplied to show that the requirements of the law are being met?

These are technically very complex questions, often with political ramifications, and Congress delegates these decisions to the regulatory agencies. What EPA does is produce fairly detailed technical rules that specify just how the regulated community will be expected to comply with the law. So regulations that are promulgated by regulatory agencies have the force of law, unlike guidelines or policies. Violators of these regulations are subject to criminal or civil penalties. EPA cannot act unless Congress has said that it can, and must act if Congress directs it to do so. Sometimes Congress stipulates a time limit and regulations must be produced quickly.

FEDERAL POLICY DECISIONS OF BIOTECHNOLOGY REGULATION

A series of federal policy decisions led to a coordinated framework for the regulation of biotechnology, which was published in June 1986 by the White House Office of Science and Technology Policy. First and probably most importantly, it was decided that products of recombinant DNA technology are not inherently more risky than those made by conventional production methods, so that no new legislation to regulate recombinant DNA products is necessary. The risks depend on hazards posed by the recipient organism and the donor gene and by the likelihood of exposure. So the decision was made to regulate the products, not the processes, of biotechnology and to do this under the currently existing regulatory authorities of different agencies.

It was also decided that risks from contained research are minimal because of limited exposure and that a scaled level of oversight is appropriate. EPA does very little regulation of laboratory research. At the greenhouse level, we might require some notification, but we do not begin to oversee biotechnology products until the point when they are released into the environment. It was also decided that the potential environmental and health benefits of recombinant DNA technology far outweigh any potential risks and that regulation should not be so burdensome as to impede the development of this promising field. Therefore, duplication of oversight by federal agencies should be avoided, not only because it would be a waste of government resources to review the same thing repeatedly, but also because it would require businesses and others to submit multiple applications for approval.

FEDERAL AGENCIES THAT REGULATE BIOTECHNOLOGY

Most of the recombinant DNA applications in the medical field (e.g., human drugs and medical diagnostic methods) are regulated by the Food and Drug Administration (FDA). People often ask me about the "flavor saver" tomato (the delayed ripening tomato in which an altered tomato gene was introduced into a tomato plant). Foods are regulated by FDA. The U.S. Department of Agriculture (USDA)—specifically the Animal and Plant Health Inspection Service in the USDA—regulates veterinary biological products, plants, and plant pests and animals or pathogens of agricultural animals. Therefore, recombinant DNA organisms that fall into any of these categories would be regulated by the USDA. EPA regulates pesticides, including those made by recombinant DNA techniques, and as a sort of catch-all, products that are not explicitly regulated by another federal agency, which includes bioremediation products.

The EPA is responsible for implementing three laws that apply to certain biotechnology products. These are the Federal Insecticide, Fungicide, and Rodenticide Act as amended, or FIFRA (P.L. 100-532, Oct. 25, 1988, 102 Stat. 2654); the Federal Food, Drug and Cosmetic Act, or FFDCA (P.L. 100-690, title II, 2403, 2631, 102 Stat. 4230, 4244); and the Toxic Substances Control Act, or TSCA (P.L. 100-551, 1, Oct. 28, 1988, 102 Stat. 2755). These laws determine what EPA can and cannot legally require.

Federal Insecticide, Fungicide, and Rodenticide Act

FIFRA regulates the marketing of pesticides, including those produced by recombinant DNA methods. It also deals with environmental release during research and development. EPA can require manufacturers to provide health and environmental effects data before a pesticide is registered for marketing in the United States, essentially to obtain a license to sell a pesticide. EPA will determine risk and specify the conditions of use—for example, the application rates and the frequency of application—and also the sites of use for the pesticide. Under FIFRA "site" has a very specific meaning. A crop (e.g., corn) is considered a site. The risks that may be posed by a pesticide used on one site, such as corn, may be quite different if the same pesticide were used on another site, such as indoors in dairy barns. Some sites will have predominantly human health risks, some will have environmental risks, some will have occupational risks, and so on.

EPA may suspend, cancel, or restrict use of a pesticide at any time if it determines that the risks outweigh the benefits of use. FIFRA is a risk-benefit balancing statute: risks from the pesticide must be balanced against the benefits of its continued use. A pesticide may pose some risk, but the benefits could be extremely high. For example, there may be a single pesticide available to treat a major pest of a major food crop, and if we cancel use of that pesticide because of risk concerns, it could result in a loss of millions of dollars to consumers because of increases in cost of food. In that case, we might decide not to cancel use of the pesticide completely, but to reduce risk by requiring other risk management methods, for example, reducing the application rate or restricting the application methods.

Federal Food, Drug and Cosmetic Act

FFDCA applies to a subset of pesticides, namely those used on food and animal feed. FFDCA directs EPA to take into account the results of toxicity testing and to estimate people's exposure to pesticides obtained in the diet. After these dietary risks are quantified, EPA does one of two things. It either sets a tolerance (an acceptable level of pesticides on food in the marketplace) or, if risk from the pesticide is considered to be negligible, it may exempt the pesticide from the requirement for a tolerance. Although the setting of tolerance levels is done by EPA, the monitoring of food for violations and the enforcement of the law is left to FDA. Most decisions regarding pesticides used on foods require an interplay between EPA and FDA. FFDCA is not a risk-benefit balancing statute, and decisions are based entirely on risk levels.

Toxic Substances Control Act

TSCA regulates the manufacture, commerce, and disposal of toxic chemicals. The concern here is not research but the entry of these products into the marketplace or the manufacturing of other products. The law authorizes EPA to screen both existing compounds and new chemicals as they are developed or brought into manufacturing processes and into commerce to identify those that are potentially dangerous. The agency has the authority to require manufacturers to provide toxicity testing information. TSCA is in a sense a risk-benefit balancing authority, because EPA must use the least burdensome risk management option to reduce risks to an acceptable level.

Many very toxic chemicals are used in manufacturing. Obviously, it is undesirable to ban these indiscriminately, but we can specify risk management methods to reduce possibilities for exposure. We can specify how chemicals will be transported and disposed of. EPA can also develop policies that promote reduced use of toxic chemicals and favor alternative environmentally friendly (or "greener") production technologies where feasible.

CONSIDERATIONS FOR DEVELOPMENT OF
REGULATORY POLICIES

How does EPA decide whether a regulatory policy needs to be developed for recombinant DNA products resulting from biotechnology? For example, do we need to modify existing regulations that were largely meant to apply to chemical compounds and in some cases to naturally occurring indigenous biocontrol agents believed to be in balance with the environment? Of course, chemical compounds are not self-reproducing so we do not have the same concerns that we might have with genetically modified organisms.

Several factors are considered in the decision to regulate. First, does the situation pose significant risk to human health or the environment? The problem with biotechnology and the release of genetically modified organisms is that nobody really knows how to quantify the risks. We cannot really say whether the risk from biotechnology is significant, but we can express concern for potential risks; until we have more experience, the thinking is that it is better for us to be on the safe side.

Second, is the situation extensive enough geographically to warrant action? If a problem is restricted to one state, it clearly does not justify the intervention of the entire federal government. However, environmental releases of genetically modified organisms from various technologies are probably occurring in all states and have been for some years, so the situation is broad enough to warrant some EPA action.

A third consideration is whether there is public concern about risks. Often scientists may not feel that public concern is justified, but the public has a right to have its needs addressed. The responses of people in various states when releases of genetically modified organisms have been planned indicate that there is some concern that these releases be of minimal risk.

Another consideration is whether industry has a need for regulations. This seems paradoxical, but companies need to be able to plan how much money they may have to spend to compile the data necessary to bring a product to the commercial stage and to register it. There is a certainty involved in knowing what the rules are instead of having decisions made on a case-by-case basis, with different reviewers making ad hoc decisions. Groups from the biotechnology industry have indicated to EPA that they would favor the development of specific guidelines or policies for recombinant DNA releases.

An important question is whether EPA has sufficient resources available to address the problem, given EPA priorities, shrinking budgets, etc. EPA is already regulating biotechnology products under the Office of Science and Technology Policy framework. By clarifying and narrowing the scope of oversight, it may be possible to reduce the resources needed to review applications and also reduce the regulatory burden on industry by screening out recombinant DNA organisms that pose minimal risks.

The final consideration is whether EPA has the statutory authority to act. Many environmental problems raise real concerns, but until Congress passes a law giving EPA authority to implement that law, we really cannot regulate. However, if biotechnology products are to be used for pesticides or if products are not regulated by another agency, EPA does have the statutory authority to regulate them.

What are the societal and economic costs of regulating, and what are the costs and benefits of not regulating? Executive orders direct EPA to consider these costs in determining whether or not to promulgate regulations although it is important to note that some environmental laws specifically prohibit this. In the case of biotechnology regulation, the societal and economic costs are probably warranted because of the need to develop a rigorous framework for risk analysis.

A CASE STUDY: RISK DETERMINATION OF TRANSGENIC PLANT PESTICIDES

A case study concerning transgenic plant pesticides illustrates some of the considerations that would be used in risk determination and how EPA policy would be applied. Some plants naturally make pesticidal substances. For example, chrysanthemums make pyrethrums, which are toxic to certain insects. Chrysanthemums are not a major component of most diets. They do not move around or contaminate the groundwater. EPA traditionally exempted plants from the requirements of FIFRA because plants are considered to be biocontrol agents and they are not considered to be very risky. However, EPA reserved the right to revoke the exemption of pesticidal plants if the situation changed enough to warrant it. Furthermore, if the pyrethrums are extracted from plants and used as active ingredients, for example, to make another pesticide that can be sprayed from a can, the pyrethrums are subject to the FIFRA requirements. If they are used on food or animal feed, they are also subject to the FFDCA requirements.

The rationale behind the earlier exemption of pesticidal plants and other biocontrol agents is that they already occur in nature. They do not expose nontarget organisms that would not otherwise be exposed, and natural cross breeding would have already occurred. However, recombinant DNA technology can now be used to construct transgenic plant pesticides, and this opens the possibility for both nontarget organisms and humans to be exposed to the pesticide by novel pathways. EPA recently developed a policy governing transgenic plant pesticides (EPA,

1994d). The level of concern for risks from transgenic plant pesticides will vary depending on the properties of both the plant and the pesticidal product.

If the plant and its progeny are contained on site, EPA would have less concern about risks than if the plant or its progeny could move off site, for example, if there were dispersal of seeds. Likewise, if pollen from the plant can be contained, there is less concern than if the pollen is not contained; it is even better if the pollen can be not made at all. If there are no weedy relatives—for example corn does not have any known relatives in the continental United States with which it can outcross—we clearly would have less concern than if a plant has many weedy relatives and can potentially outcross and spread the transgenic gene into the wild.

Different risk concerns are associated with pesticidal products. Pesticidal products such as pyrethrum, for example, that are normally a component of the plant or of a cross-hybridizing species into which the pesticide gene is introduced, would cause much less concern than one that was not normally a component of the plant and would not be likely to get into it by traditional breeding methods. A pesticidal product that readily degrades in the environment is of less concern than one that is highly persistent and for which exposure will continue over time. A pesticidal product that may act by a nontoxic mode of action—for example, a structural modification that may make it more difficult for an insect to penetrate the cuticle of the plant—would certainly be of less concern than a pesticide that acts directly by a toxic mechanism on the target pest, because of the possibility of lack of specificity and toxic effects on nontarget organisms. Another factor is the level of exposure. A pesticide that might be used in a greenhouse situation only, for example in nurseries, would be of less concern than a pesticidal gene introduced into a food or feed crop, particularly a major crop such as corn, which occupies about 71 million acres (USDA, 1993).

DEVELOPING EPA REGULATIONS

How then does EPA develop environmental regulations such as those now under development for transgenic plant pesticides? Although many people are not aware of it, opportunities exist at many levels for input by other agencies, other EPA offices, and nongovernmental groups. Everything is done in a public forum. The development of regulations involves resolving the interests of conflicting groups.

Figure 21-1 shows the developmental pathway for a biotechnology regulation. Within EPA, the development of the regulations and the wording of the text is guided by a work group headed by the office that is responsible for implementing the law in question. EPA recently stream-

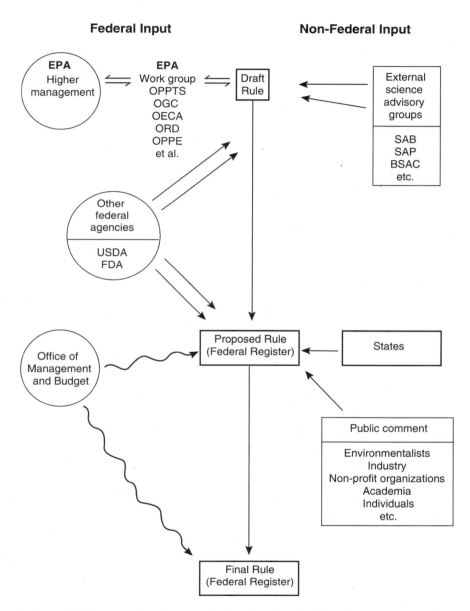

FIGURE 21-1 Biotechnology regulation: developmental pathway.

lined the regulatory and policy development process. Tiered levels of across-office participation and senior management involvement are scaled to reflect the proposed action's environmental and economic significance, external stakeholders' interest in it, its cross-media or cross-office consequences, and its precedent-setting nature. The work-group process applies to development of policies and regulations belonging to the two highest tiers [Administrator's priority actions and cross-agency actions (EPA, 1994a)]. Both TSCA and FIFRA fall within the purview of the Office of Prevention, Pesticides, and Toxic Substances, which provides much of the expertise on exposure pathways, risk analysis, and scientific issues.

The program office generally is concerned with regulatory clarity and risk management. If a regulation is presented clearly, the regulated community can read it and know right away if talks with EPA are needed about a product. A carefully defined scope of regulation will focus examination on those products that are believed to pose the greatest risk and will exclude or exempt from coverage those posing negligible risk. The program office assesses the level of risk posed by a situation and develops several options for managing the risk.

Representatives from other EPA offices also serve on the work group. The Office of General Counsel has to defend EPA in court when the agency is sued. EPA is sued regularly both by industry and environmentalists. The environmentalists usually accuse EPA of not doing enough to protect the public, and industry usually accuses us of overstepping our authority and overregulating. The Office of General Counsel is very concerned about whether the law actually gives EPA the authority to require people in the regulated community to take a specific action. They want to be sure that the regulation will stand up to legal challenge.

Representatives from the Office of Enforcement and Compliance Assurance (OECA), which goes after violators of regulations, are also on the work group. OCEA is generally eager to have rules written that permit EPA to detect violations and, if necessary, impose clean-up costs and penalties.

The Office of Research and Development reviews the scientific basis of the proposed regulation and offers advice on how risk is determined. Risk assessment is a very controversial area. There is not always agreement on how to quantify risks or what constitutes a risk.

My office, the Office of Policy, Planning and Evaluation (OPPE), is interested in seeing that the rules will promote the overall goals of EPA and that all EPA program offices speak with one voice. This is important because, besides the laws I have mentioned here, EPA through other program offices issues regulations under other acts. OPPE wants to be sure that we do not just transfer a problem from one medium to another. For example, we do not want to take an air pollution problem, write a regulation about air, and have the same pollutant now show up in solid waste. We also want the regulation to be cost effective and risk based.

All the offices work out the details of a draft rule. At various decision points, or if there are disagreements, senior management is consulted to select among various risk management options. Various external science advisory groups may provide input on key scientific issues during the development process. Senior management also takes into account political and economic considerations, for example, whether the burden of risks or the costs of compliance may fall on a tiny segment of the affected community. Eventually the offices concur on an acceptable draft rule. Reviewing bodies include, but are not limited to, the Science Advisory Board, the Science Advisory Panel (which is specific for pesticides), the Biotechnology Science Advisory Council, and others. We solicit opinions from the National Research Council, the Institutes of Medicine, and other bodies.

After we take the comments of the scientific reviewers into account and modify the draft rule, we consult other federal agencies. I mentioned that there is some overlap with USDA and FDA. These agencies have to be satisfied that what EPA proposes is not going to conflict with what they have to do. Finally, when all the offices have signed off on the rule and the EPA administrator has approved it, the rule goes to the Office of Management and Budget (OMB) in the White House. That office has to ensure that the rule concurs with various executive orders (e.g., Executive Order 12866, which mandates cost-benefit analyses for major actions or those that affect the economy, and Executive Order 12898, which addresses environmental justice in minority and low-income populations) and that all affected agencies involved are satisfied. Then the rule is published in the Federal Register, usually as a proposed rule.

This is where the public becomes involved, if they have not already served on one of the science advisory groups. EPA is required to request and to consider public comment on proposed rules, and we receive public comment from environmental groups, industry, states, community groups, academia, and private individuals. So if there is a regulation that may affect how you do business or may have a bearing on your life, you definitely have the right—indeed, you are expected—to contact the appropriate agency and say whether or not you think the regulation is a good idea and your reasons for thinking this.

After the 90-day comment period closes, all comments are analyzed, summarized, and taken into account in the promulgation of the final rule. If public comment is overwhelmingly opposed to a proposed rule and we are fairly certain that the public comment is representative, we have two choices. Either we can go ahead with the rule knowing that it is going to cause a great deal of political flak (usually the higher management will take that route only if they can be convinced that there is a very good reason), or we can conclude that our proposed ideas were bad and go back to the early stage of the process. Because of the extensive pre-publication consultations, this does not happen too often, but when it does, the proposed rule is modified on the basis of public comment. Again we will get input from other agencies and OMB will review the rule. After OMB approves it, it is published as a final rule in the *Federal Register*, at which time it has the force of law.

REGULATIONS FOR BIOTECHNOLOGY PRODUCTS

Three EPA regulations that apply to biotechnology products were recently published. The first of the rules comes under FIFRA and concerns microbial pesticides, including those genetically modified, and non-indigenous microorganisms (EPA, 1994c). The second rule regulates transgenic plant pesticides under FIFRA and FFDCA (EPA, 1994e). The third rule, concerning microbial products of biotechnology, comes under TSCA and applies to bioremediation agents and other non-food, non-pesticide products (EPA, 1994b).

ROLE OF BIOTECHNOLOGY IN POLLUTION PREVENTION

What biotechnology products do we see on the horizon? I think the most exciting possibilities are those relating to waste management strategies. "Waste" is really another way of saying pollution. For example, a highly toxic chemical that may be safely used in manufacturing can cause problems if it gets out into the environment. This is both pollution and a waste of resources.

The waste management strategies developed to deal with pollution are remediation, waste conversion, and pollution prevention. The least desirable is remediation, because this occurs after the damage is done. However, we definitely need remediation products, and we are counting on biotechnology to give them to us. Somewhat earlier in the waste pipeline is waste conversion. In this strategy, waste—that is, toxic pollutants—are converted into harmless by-products or, if possible, useful products. Rarely are these kinds of strategies 100 percent effective and they also occur after the pollutant has been produced.

Probably the most effective strategy is pollution prevention. This means altering the manufacturing process so that waste is not produced. Most biotechnology products near the commercialization stage are biopesticides, and the focus of biopesticides is pollution prevention.

Biopesticides create safer pesticides that can decrease the use of conventional toxic chemical pesticides and their release into the environment. Two applications for which we now have regulations in place are microbial pesticides and plant pesticides. With microbial pesticides, microorganisms that are pest-specific pathogens are genetically engineered so that they have enhanced or in some cases new pesticidal properties. If they are pest specific, the risk to nontarget organisms and to humans is much less than with conventional pesticides, some of which act by highly toxic actions analogous to nerve gas.

The second application is the plant pesticide. Plants can be genetically engineered to be pest resistant or to express pesticidal substances directly. Again, there is no waste because all the pesticide is in the plant. There is no worry about spraying nontarget organisms in the area or about the pesticide moving off site and contaminating groundwater or about other environmental concerns arising from the use of chemical pesticides.

Bioprocessing and bioremediation have significant potential for pollution prevention and environmental remediation. Bioprocessing and bioremediation agents are primarily in the research stage, but we hope to see commercial applications in the future because they provide opportunities to solve very important environmental problems. For example, microbes, plants, and fungi could be modified to synthesize polymers used in plastics, paint, and adhesive manufacturing. Traditional manufacturing processes generate many toxic by-products. If these polymers could be generated biosynthetically, toxic waste generation would be reduced at the source.

As far as waste conversion is concerned, the possibility exists to convert organic wastes, such as those from sludge and from water purification plants, into methane or alcohol. These products could be used instead of fossil fuels, sparing them for manufacturing uses where there are no substitutes.

Remediation is clearly of great interest to EPA because of the halogenated organic compounds that have persisted in the environment, as well as heavy metals. It is very striking that in the 1970s EPA canceled all uses of the pesticide dichlorodiphenyl-trichloroethane (DDT) and all manufacturing and most uses of polychlorinated biphenyls (PCBs) (EPA, 1972, 1979). Yet in a 1990 survey of fish tissues in the United States, the most predominant contaminants in fish tissues were PCBs and dichloro-diphenyl-dichloroethylene (DDE), a breakdown product of DDT that is highly toxic in its own right (EPA, 1992). EPA has done all that it can to stop the introduction of these chemicals into the environment, but because of their persistence they are continuing to pose a problem that may only be resolved by remediation.

CONCLUSION

Environmental applications of biotechnology have brought us to the threshold of commercialization of many products, primarily biopesticides. These products may soon enable us to stop or in some cases reverse the negative effects of human activities on the environment. Initially some in the biotechnology community may feel that federal regulators are guarding the door to the marketplace too vigilantly in the face of what many view as largely theoretical risks. However, public concerns about the safety of this relatively new technology must be addressed by a rigorous and credible oversight process, at least until biotechnology gains wider public acceptance and people are more comfortable with its use.

What we do not want to happen to this promising industry is, through sloppy regulation, for a risky product to get out into the environment and cause a disaster. This would give the entire industry a black eye. As an analogy, consider what happened when the Hindenburg exploded. We do not want the dirigible industry to be a model for the biotechnology industry.

In the future, as we gain more experience about the survival and dispersal of cloned genetic information and as we get more information about the level of perturbation that can be expected in ecosystems in which new organisms are introduced, we will likely see exclusions from regulation for classes of genetically modified organisms that have been determined empirically to pose minimal risks. As we build up a larger database that allows us to make more accurate risk assessments, streamlined risk-based determinations will very likely become commonplace for most recombinant DNA products.

REFERENCES

U.S. Department of Agriculture. 1993. Agricultural Chemical Usage: 1992 Field Crops Summary. Washington, DC: USDA National Agricultural Statistics Service.

U.S. Environmental Protection Agency. 1972. Consolidated DDT hearings opinion and order of the administrator. Fed. Regist. 37 (131):13369-13376.

U.S. Environmental Protection Agency. 1979. Polychlorinated biphenyls (PCBs) manufacturing, processing, distribution in commerce, and use prohibitions: final rule. Fed. Regist. 44 (106): 31514-31568.

U.S. Environmental Protection Agency. 1992. National Study of Chemical Residues in Fish. Vol. I. EPA 823-R-92-008a. Washington, DC: Office of Science and Technology.

U.S. Environmental Protection Agency. 1994a. Initiation of EPA's New Regulatory and Policy Development Process. Memorandum from the administrator to EPA's assistant administrators, general counsel, associate administrator, regional administrators, and office directors.

U.S. Environmental Protection Agency. 1994b. 40CFR Part 700, et al. Microbial products of biotechnology; proposed regulation under the Toxic Substances Control Act; proposed rule. Fed. Regist. 59 (169):45526-45585.

U.S. Environmental Protection Agency. 1994c. 40CFR Part 172. Microbial pesticides; experimental use permits and notifications; final rule. Fed. Regist. 59 (169):45600-45615.

U.S. Environmental Protection Agency. 1994d. Plant-pesticides subject to the Federal Insecticide, Fungicide, and Rodenticide Act (FIFRA) and the Federal Food, Drug and Cosmetic Act (FFDCA); proposed policy; notice. Fed. Regist. 59 (225):60496-60518.

U.S. Environmental Protection Agency. 1994e. 40 CFR Parts 152, 174, and 180. Proposed exemptions from the requirement of a tolerance for plant pesticides and nucleic acids and viral coat proteins produced in plants under FFDCA, and plant-pesticides subject to FIFRA; proposed rules. Fed. Regist. 59 (225):60519-60547.

Biographies of the Contributors

Ruth Ellen Bulger is vice president for scientific affairs, Henry M. Jackson Foundation for the Advancement of Military Medicine, Rockville, Maryland. Before assuming that position in 1993, she was director, Division of Health Sciences Policy, Institute of Medicine, National Academy of Sciences, Washington, D.C. From 1978 to 1988, she was professor in the graduate school of biomedical sciences at the University of Texas Health Sciences Center, Houston. She is the co-editor of *The Ethical Dimensions of the Biological Sciences* (1993) and supervised or helped prepare approximately 40 studies at the Institute of Medicine, including several on women's health. She holds a Ph.D. in anatomy from the University of Washington.

C. Thomas Caskey is Senior Vice President of Research at Merck Research Laboratories, West Point since January 1, 1995. Prior to his departure from Baylor College of Medicine in Houston, he served as chairman of the Department of Molecular and Human Genetics, director of Baylor's Human Genome Center and an investigator with Howard Hughes Medical Institute. He is also president of the international Human Genome Organization, an organization of scientists involved in the Human Genome Project. A member of the National Academy of Sciences, Dr. Caskey received his medical degree from Duke University Medical School and did postdoctoral work in genetics at the National Heart and Lung Institute, National Institutes of Health.

Rebecca S. Eisenberg is professor of law at the University of Michigan Law School, Ann Arbor, where she has taught courses in intellectual property, protection of technology, trademarks and unfair competition, and legal issues in scientific research. She received a J.D. degree from the University of California, Berkeley, School of Law. She has lectured and written on patent rights in the Human Genome Project, has a grant from the Department of Energy to study the role of patents in technology transfer in the Human Genome Project, and is a member of the National Institutes of Health–Department of Energy Working Group on the Ethical, Legal, and Social Implications of Human Genome Research.

Suzanne Giannini Spohn is senior scientist at the U.S. Environmental Protection Agency (EPA) in the Office of Policy, Planning and Evaluation. Her areas of expertise include microbiology and parasitology. She has done extensive research in the field of communicable diseases. She is a member of EPA's Risk Assessment Forum and Cancer Risk Assessment Group. Before going to EPA, Dr. Giannini Spohn was a full-time member of the faculty at the University of Maryland Medical School, where she holds an appointment as adjunct associate professor.

M. R. C. Greenwood was associate director for science, White House Office of Science and Technology Policy when she and Rachel Levinson coauthored this chapter. She has since returned to the position of dean of graduate studies and vice provost for academic research at the University of California, Davis. She is also professor in the departments of nutrition and internal medicine. Her research interests are in developmental cell biology, genetics, physiology, and nutrition. Dr. Greenwood's work over the past 25 years, focusing on the genetic causes of obesity, is recognized worldwide. In 1992, she was elected to the Institute of Medicine of the National Academy of Sciences.

Daniel E. Koshland, Jr., is professor emeritus of molecular biology at the University of California, Berkeley, and was the long-time editor-in-chief of *Science* magazine until recently. He helped establish and was chairman of the Academy Forum, a committee of the National Academy of Sciences that is charged with helping to develop policy on issues that pose dilemmas at the interface between science and societal problems. Dr. Koshland's research has produced major advances in the understanding of enzymes and protein chemistry. He is an international leader in research on short- and long-term memory. His awards include the National Medal of Science, the Pauling Award of the American Chemical Society, and election to the National Academy of Sciences.

Neal F. Lane is director of the National Science Foundation, an independent agency of the federal government that provides support for research and education in science, mathematics, and engineering. Before becoming NSF director in October 1993, Dr. Lane was provost and professor of physics at Rice University. He is the former chancellor of the University of Colorado at Colorado Springs and former director of the Division of Physics of the National Science Foundation. Dr. Lane has authored or co-authored more than 90 scientific papers and publications, including a textbook on quantum physics. He is a fellow of the American Physical Society and of the American Association for the Advancement of Science.

Louis Lasagna is dean of the Sackler School of Graduate Biomedical Sciences, Tufts University, Boston. He is also academic dean at the school of medicine, professor of psychiatry, and professor of pharmacology. He has served on or consulted with numerous government agencies and committees, including the U.S. Department of Health and Human Services Advisory Committee on the Food and Drug Administration and the National Committee to Review Current Procedures for Approval of New Drugs for Cancer and AIDS. His many honors include the J. Allyn Taylor International Prize in Medicine in 1993.

Rachel E. Levinson is the assistant director for life sciences, White House Office of Science and Technology Policy. Ms. Levinson is on detail from the Office of the Director, National Institutes of Health, where she was involved in policy issues related to biotechnology and technology transfer, oversight of recombinant DNA research, and initiation of the NIH Human Genome Project. From 1973 until 1983, Ms. Levinson was in the National Cancer Institute intramural research program where her work focused on glycoproteins and structural proteins associated with cancer.

Kathleen S. Matthews is Harry C. and Olga K. Weiss Professor of Biochemistry & Cell Biology at Rice University and was chair of the department from 1987 to 1995. Her major research interests are chemistry and molecular biology of proteins; studies on DNA regulatory proteins employing chemical modification, genetic modification, spectroscopy, and other physical methods. She has been a member of the advisory committee to NIH, NSF, HHMI, and the state of Texas and is associate editor of the *Journal of Biological Chemistry*. She holds a Ph.D. in biochemistry from the University of California, Berkeley.

Larry V. McIntire is the E. D. Butcher Professor of Chemical and Biomedical Engineering at Rice University. He is also chair of the Institute of Biosciences and Bioengineering and director of the Cox Laboratory for

Biomedical Engineering within the Institute. His research interests include the effects of flow on mammalian-cell metabolism, molecular mechanisms of cell adhesion, tissue engineering, mammalian-cell culture, and bioengineering aspects of vascular biology. Dr. McIntire is the recipient of a National Institutes of Health MERIT award and is a founding fellow of the American Institute of Medical and Biological Engineering.

Barbara Mishkin is an attorney who concentrates on health regulatory issues, particularly the federal regulation of biomedical research, scientific misconduct, institutional and medical staff bylaws, and the credentialing and disciplining of practitioners. Before joining Hogan & Hartson in 1983, Ms. Mishkin served as deputy director of the President's Commission for the Study of Ethical Problems in Medicine and Biomedical and Behavioral Research. She was previously staff director, U.S. Department of Health, Education, and Welfare Ethics Advisory Board.

Robert M. Nerem is institute professor and Parker H. Petit Distinguished Chair for Engineering in Medicine, George Woodruff School of Mechanical Engineering, Georgia Institute of Technology, Atlanta. Dr. Nerem is president of the International Union for Physical and Engineering Sciences in Medicine and immediate past president of the International Federation for Medical and Biological Engineering. He is the president of the newly established American Institute of Medical and Biological Engineering. In 1988, Professor Nerem was elected to the National Academy of Engineering and in 1992, to the Institute of Medicine of the National Academy of Sciences. Research interests include biofluid mechanics, cardiovascular devices, cellular engineering, vascular biology, atherosclerosis, and tissue engineering.

Gene F. Parkin is professor and chair of the Department of Civil and Environmental Engineering at the University of Iowa. He is director of the Center for Health Effects of Environmental Contamination and serves on the executive committee of the Center for Biocatalysis and Bioprocessing. He holds a Ph.D. degree in environmental engineering from Stanford University. His teaching interests have been in biological treatment processes and environmental chemistry. His research has been directed toward anaerobic biological processes and bioremediation of waters contaminated with organic chemicals.

Mark Rothstein is Law Foundation Professor of Law and director of the Health Law and Policy Institute at the University of Houston. He has concentrated his research on employment and occupational health law. He has written on a wide range of issues, including bioethics, disabilities law, drug abuse, employment law, genetics, health policy, and occupation health. He has served as a consultant or adviser to the Department of Energy, the Office of Technology Assessment of the U.S. Congress, the American Medical Association, the National Center for Human Genome Research, and the Institute of Medicine of the National Academy of Sciences.

Frederick B. Rudolph is professor and chair of Biochemistry & Cell Biology at Rice University. He is also executive director of the Institute of Biosciences and Bioengineering and director of the Mabee Laboratory for Biochemical and Genetic Engineering within the institute. His research interests include factors and mechanisms involved in the control of metabolism, protein structure and function, regulation and control of nucleotide metabolism, new techniques in enzyme purification, effect of dietary nucleotides on immune function and tumor growth, and solvent production by bacterial fermentations.

Jerome Schultz has been director of the Center for Biotechnology and Bioengineering at the University of Pittsburgh since its inception in 1987. Professor Schultz served with the National Science Foundation as Deputy Director for Cross-Disciplinary Research. In that capacity, he contributed to the development of the foundation's Engineering Research Center Program and was responsible of the development of programs in emerging engineering technologies such as biotechnology, bioengineering, and lightwave technology. After receiving his Ph.D. degree in biochemistry from the University of Wisconsin, he worked for Lederle Laboratories developing antibiotics, enzymes, and steroids.

Michael L. Shuler is Samuel B. Eckert Professor of Chemical Engineering with joint appointment in the Institute of Food Science at Cornell University. He holds a Ph.D. in chemical engineering from the University of Minnesota. His research interests in biochemical engineering include the areas of growth characteristics and product formation from plant cell tissue cultures, the development and experimental verification of models for the growth of individual cells, and the response of natural ecosystems to toxic chemicals and biodegradation.

Anna Marie Skalka is scientific director of the Institute for Cancer Research and vice president of the Fox Chase Cancer Center in Philadelphia. Before assuming that position, she was head of the Department of Molecular Oncology at the Roche Institute of Molecular Biology, Nutley, New Jersey. She holds a Ph.D. in microbiology from New York University.

Judith P. Swazey is president of The Acadia Institute, a nonprofit center in Bar Harbor, Maine, that does research, consults, and develops educational programs dealing with issues concerning medicine, science, and society. Dr. Swazey, who received her Ph.D. in the history of science from Harvard University, also is an adjunct professor of social and behavioral sciences at Boston University Schools of Medicine and Public Health. Her work has focused on social, ethical, legal, and policy aspects of biomedical research and health care, professional ethics, and issues in graduate and professional education. She currently is principal investigator of the institute's study of professional values and ethical issues in the graduate education of scientists and engineers.

Eric Tomlinson is president and chief executive officer of GENEMEDICINE, INC., a biotechnology company based in The Woodlands, Texas, developing controllable gene therapy products for direct administration to patients. From 1984 to January 1990, he was worldwide head of advanced drug delivery research for Ciba-Geigy Pharmaceuticals with responsibility for creating and leading its multidisciplinary research and development program in site-specific (protein) drug delivery. He has authored or co-authored more than 200 scientific publications and articles in the pharmaceutical sciences. He received his doctor of science degree from the University of London. He is a fellow of the Royal Pharmaceutical Society of Great Britain, awarded for distinction in the science of pharmacy.

José E. Trías was vice president and general counsel of the Howard Hughes Medical Institute (HHMI) in Chevy Chase, Maryland, the largest private philanthropic biomedical research organization in the United States. HHMI's scientific, legal and administrative staff oversees implementation of the organization's policies on research integrity. A graduate of Yale Law School, Mr. Trías was the author of a report on human rights in Chile and served on the advisory board of the International Human Rights, Trial Observer Project of the American Bar Association. He had been the vice chairman of the Puerto Rican Legal Defense and Education Fund.

Alexander Wlodawer is director of the Macromolecular Structure Laboratory of the Frederick Cancer Research and Development Center, National Cancer Institute, Frederick, Maryland. He received his Ph.D. in molecular biology from the University of California, Los Angeles, with specialization in crystallography. He held appointments in Warsaw and Rome, at Stanford University, and at the National Bureau of Standards before joining the National Cancer Institute in 1987. He has wide interests in biophysical research and is on the board of *Protein Science* journal.

Savio Lau-Ching Woo is a professor of cell biology, molecular genetics, and pediatrics at Baylor College of Medicine. He is also director of the Center for Gene Therapy at Baylor and an investigator with the Howard Hughes Medical Institute. He is a member of the Human Genome Organization, the American College of Medical Genetics, and the board of Scientific Counselors for the National Institute of Child Health and Human Development. Dr. Woo was recently elected to the board of directors for the American Society of Human Genetics.

Index

G

β-Galactosidase, 77-78, 80
Ganciclovir, in gene therapy, 81-86
Gaucher's disease, 66
Gene therapy
  adenoviral vector delivery
    systems, 77-86
  anti-cancer, 23
  applications, 23, 54-55, 61-62, 68,
    86
  for brain tumors, 85-86
  delivery systems, 69-70, 71, 72, 74-
    86, 88, 89
  ex vivo strategy, 72-74
  for immunodeficiency diseases,
    68-69
  for neurological disorders, 86-87,
    91
  plasmid DNA in, 69-70
  process, 68-69
  prospects for, 61, 65-66, 70-71
  regulation of expression, 72
  research origins, 64-65
  retrovirus delivery system, 74-77
  for solid tumors, 81-85
  source genes, 72
  technical basis, 68
  tissue engineering for delivery
    systems, 88, 97
  in vivo strategy, 74
General Agreement on Tariffs and
  Trade, 231
Genetic risk, *vi*
  diagnostic procedures, 49-50
  diseases associated with, 68
  epigenetic model, 104
  insurance practice and, 194-195,
    206
  possibilities for disease
    prevention, 50-51, 193
  privacy issues, 51-53, 203-204, 206
  trinucleotide repeat diseases, 46-49
  workplace discrimination and, 206
Genetic science
  cloning, 195-196
  drug production, 53-54

early DNA research, 3-4
effects on social attitudes and
  behavior, 205
genetic enhancement, 202
near-term ethical issues, 205-207
tissue engineering and, 97
understanding of plant biology,
  108
Genetic screening
  access, 201-202, 206
  for behavioral traits, 203
  for colon cancer, 19
  effects on interpersonal relations,
    202
  implications for people existing
    with disorders, 202
Genome mapping
  basics, 13
  microbiological research, 15-17
  research development, 44-46
  similarity among organisms, 13
Glucocerebrosidase, 66
Government interventions/policy
  allocation of research resources,
    218-220
  authority for biotechnology
    regulation, 248-249
  in biotechnology, *vii*, 223-224, 247,
    256
  case study, 251-252
  drug development, international
    comparison of, 223, 225-226
  drug pricing and reimbursement,
    228-230
  federal research budget, 233-236,
    241
  future prospects, 258
  human subjects research, 214-216,
    217-218
  interagency efforts, 255
  international agreements, 227-228
  investigating and sanctioning
    scientific misconduct, 184-190
  investment in biotechnology, 241-
    244
  limitations of law, 246-247

drug pricing and reimbursement,
228-230
patent system, 162, 165, 230-231

J

Japan, 225-226, 227, 229-230

L

Life expectancy, 193-194
Ligase enzyme, 11
Liver
bioartificial, 91-92
gene therapy, 72-73, 76-77, 78-79
Lung cancer, 107

M

Machado-Joseph disease, 49
Malpractice, 217
Massachusetts Institute of
Technology, 135-136
Mathematical modeling, 106
Medical science, *vi*, 17
change vs. progress in, 210-211
contributions of Howard Hughes
Medical Institute, 156-157
diagnostic imaging technology, 66
DNA-based diagnostic
techniques, 43, 49-50
genetic diagnostic testing, 49-50
genetic science for disease
prevention, 50-51
Human Genome Project in, 46, 50
patient decision-making and, 212
research on women's health
issues, 208-209
Metabolic control theory, 103-104
Microcephalic infants, 196-197
Molecular cell biology
AIDS/HIV research, 24-26
biomaterials development, 96-97
in bioremediation, 126
of cancer, 17-19
cancer treatment, 19-23

limitations of research, 16
mathematical modeling, 106
prospects for technical
development, 26
research contributions, 15-16, 64
technical advances, 16-17, 64
vascular system mechanical
environment, 92-94
Mutations
in cancer, 17, 105
in colon cancer, 18-19
diagnostic screening, 49-50
DNA in, 6-7
in HIV virus, 24, 26
trinucleotide repeats, 47-49
Myocardial infarction, 66, 92
Myoscint, 66
Myotonic dystrophy, 47-49

N

National Institute for Standards and
Technology, 242
National Institutes of Health
applications for cDNA patents,
167-170
biotechnology industry
collaborations, 243
funding trends, 153
research guidelines, 12-13, 188,
189, 213, 219
National Research Council, 136
National Science and Technology
Council, 241
National Science Foundation, 137, 140-
141
on academic-industry
collaboration, 147-151
centers for academic-industry
collaboration, 148-149
on patents, 150
on technology transfer, 150
Neurological disorders, gene therapy
for, 86-87, 91
NIH. *See* National Institutes of Health